HOLISTIC
WOMAN'S HERBAL

HOLISTIC
WOMAN'S HERBAL

---

*How to Achieve Health
and Well-being at Any Age*

BY KITTY CAMPION

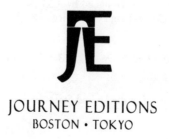

JOURNEY EDITIONS
BOSTON • TOKYO

This book presents information and material about holistic herbal treatments. This book is intended to supplement, and not replace, treatment by a physician or other licensed medical practitioner. Consult your health care provider before adopting any of the holistic treatments described herein. The adoption and application of the material offered in this book is at the reader's discretion and sole responsibility. The author and publisher of this book are not responsible in any manner whatsoever for any injury that may occur indirectly or directly from the use of this book.

First published in the United States of America in 1996 by
JOURNEY EDITIONS
an imprint of Charles E. Tuttle Co., Inc. of Rutland, Vermont, and Tokyo, Japan,
with editorial offices at
153 Milk Street
Boston, Massachusetts 02109

Library of Congress Cataloging-in-Publication Data

Campion, Kitty.
    Holistic woman's herbal : how to achieve health and well-being at
any age / by Kitty Campion.
        p. cm.
Includes bibliographical references and index.
ISBN 1-885203-37-3
    1. Herbs—Therapeutic use. 2. Women—Health and hygiene.
3. Holistic medicine. I. Title.
RM666.H33C3635 1996
615' .321.' 082—dc20   96–18750
                                       CIP

Designed by AB3
Cover design by Kathryn Sky-Peck

01 00 99 98 97 96   1 3 5 7 9 10 8 6 4 2

Printed in the United States of America

• DEDICATION •

To all my one-winged angels:
Clive and Margaret, Pam and Rod, Sandy and Liz.

We are each of us angels
With only one wing.
And we can fly only
by embracing
each other

LUCIANO de CRESCENZO

ACKNOWLEDGEMENTS

My grateful thanks for the tenacity of my literary agent Susan Mears, who sold a trilogy to Bloomsbury, of which this is the first volume. Rowena Gaunt was clear-sighted enough to accept the proposition and her input has been immensely practical. Sandy Williams, my personal assistant, knows this manuscript as well as I do because she typed every word of it with cheerfulness and amazing speed. I was given sanctuary by the superb staff at Rookery Hall in Nantwich and by the Stakis Hotel in Stoke-on-Trent, so that I could escape my normal busy life and write in an oasis of peace and calm. Richard Schulze gave me permission to quote several of his magnificent formulations in this book and I have been particularly inspired by the pioneering work of Lynn McTaggart, the Editor of *What Doctors Don't Tell You*. The extracts on pages 117 and 142 are from *Everywoman's Book*, Paavo Airola, Health Plus Publishers, Phoenix, Arizona, USA, 1979.

FOREWORD

It is almost twenty years since I first heard of Kitty Campion, her work and her writings. Her writings very much appealed to me as they showed a lot of common sense. I really wanted to meet this lady and I was lucky enough that one day a very well-known politician picked her book out of my book case and asked if I knew her. I told him that I didn't, but it turned out that he was equally keen to meet Kitty. I searched for her home address and finally found it.

I was even more fortunate that Kitty came up to visit my clinic in Scotland. We had a very interesting and most worthwhile conversation, and I discovered that Kitty had a very rich knowledge of herbal medicine. On top of this, she knew a lot about diet and lifestyle. I invited her to stay over, and the next day we talked and talked, and talked, and kept talking!

Our friendship has been of great mutual benefit. I encouraged her at great length and told her that although she was an excellent author – much better than myself – she had also been gifted with a greater talent for helping people. In fact, I almost had to force her to give up some of her business life and travelling so that she could devote more of her life to helping people. Kitty showed a great compassion, not only for people, but also for animals. She also possessed a great knowledge of food and food combining, energy, the future of medicine, and deeply believed that nature is the best healer we have.

I was very happy to know that she took my advice, started studying and has since treated hundreds of people with great success. Some patients who we have treated together always spoke about her with great admiration, as well as with a lot of gratitude and happiness for the hard work and effort that she put into relieving their different complaints.

I strongly stress in every lecture that man does not have one body but three bodies – the physical, the mental and emotional. Kitty has come through a lot in life and has learned to know the harmonies existing between the mind, body and spirit. She especially understands the problems that women can go through in life. Her books on women's complaints are outstanding, and from the hundreds of books for women on the mind, body and spirit, Kitty's books show the tremendous understanding that she has developed over the years.

I was greatly honoured to be asked to do the foreword for this excellent and comprehensive book which covers everything a woman needs to know in looking after herself. Kitty has used both intuition and research. One can see how much time and effort has gone into *Holistic Woman's Herbal* and it makes for most interesting reading.

Today in this atomic, nuclear, scientific age, medicine has become so complicated. One doesn't really know what to take and how safe it actually is. Kitty leads the way with sensible advice on home methods and herbal remedies which can often take the place of pharmaceutical products with their side effects and unknown outcomes. This book shows the author's terrific knowledge of nature and all that nature has to offer. Her experience from world travels, as well as feedback from her patients, show how readers can help themselves to better health.

Jan de Vries
D.Ho.med., D.O., M.R.O., N.D., M.R.N.D.Ac., M.B.Ac.A.

CONTENTS

CHAPTER 1:

THE ADVANTAGES OF HERBALISM

———

In 1974 following a worldwide study by two international health agencies, the Director General of the World Health Organisation (WHO) pronounced that Western methods of medicine could not be used alone if the world were to achieve an adequate standard of health care before the dawning of the next century. Every country of the world is represented in the World Health Assembly and all are united in their endorsement of the traditional medical systems of their countries, most of which depend heavily on herbs. Developing countries simply don't have the financial resources to pay for Western style technological medicine.

The cost of allopathic health care in the West is rocketing. The British National Health Service (NHS) limps from one financial crisis to another and the burgeoning cost of health care in the United States (US) is a major political issue. None of this would matter if the sums spent bought higher standards of health to the Western world. After all, as my patients frequently observe, what is life worth if you don't have that basic prerequisite – good health? But in the US life expectancy for men and women of all ages is actually falling and infant mortality is on the increase in many developed countries. In Britain the number of babies born congenitally malformed or who grow up educationally subnormal has been rising steadily since the late-1940s. The figures for degenerative diseases such as arthritis, cancer and diabetes show no sign of decline and Britain has the highest heart death rate in the world as well as the worst infant mortality figures in Europe. Indeed the shocking fact is that after the age of forty-five Britain's life expectancy is among the lowest of any developed country.

• IATROGENIC DISEASE •

Iatrogenic disease, caused by medical examination or treatment, is on the increase. Each year, people die following operations which were probably not strictly necessary. In the UK one in six hospital beds is currently taken up by those suffering from adverse reactions to chemical drugs.

Unsurprisingly, people are flocking back to traditional medicine and words like 'country goodness', 'wholesome' and 'natural' are so overused by marketeers they are becoming meaningless. But before herbal medicine is wrongly elevated to the status of a universal panacea, I should point out that it is the chemical bastardisation of the properties of herbs that has, in many instances, led to iatrogenic disease in the first place. Many people fail to realise that conventional medicine is in fact firmly rooted in herbalism. They tend to assume, if they think about it at all, that all those multi-coloured tablets have nothing to do with nature, whereas medical science still depends strongly on plant life to provide the blueprint for much modern medicine. Pharmacy tends to be more reliable because it enables chemicals to be reproduced in accurate doses and, given the correct storage conditions, such medicines remain effective over time. But the advantages of science are limited. It is the pharmacologist's concern to extract the exact chemical from a plant which will cure a specific disease, and these chemicals tend to be very potent simply because they are so concentrated. Once inside the body they have an ungovernable habit of travelling to parts they are not supposed to be treating, giving rise to iatrogenic disease.

• HERBAL MEDICINE V. CONVENTIONAL DRUGS •

It is here that the herbalist's use of the whole herb rather than simply a few of its concentrated chemical constituents comes into its own, for the use of the whole plant, balanced as it is by many other constituents, is altogether milder and more gentle, avoiding the toxic side-effects of its chemical cousins. The herb *Ephedra Sinensis* (not to be muddled with the American species of ephedra called 'desert tea') is a good example. It is a natural source of the drug ephedrine which is used to help asthmatics, but used in this form it also raises the blood pressure. Fortunately, the plant itself contains norephedrine and pseud-ephedrine which have a slightly antagonistic affect to ephedrine, so buffering its action. Thus asthma can be helped using a remedy based on the whole plant without upsetting the patient's blood pressure. The Chinese have used ephedra, known to them as *Ma huang*, for centuries for precisely this purpose.

As a herbalist I have a quarrel with allopathic medicine which disturbs me even more. Drugs are merely suppressive. They are not designed to restore general health or even to encourage the body's natural healing process. Discomfort escalating into pain is the body's own alarm system to let you know something is wrong and needs immediate attention. Ignoring it, blocking or suppressing it seems to me to be as ludicrous as being woken by the sound of a smoke alarm, only to get out of bed, tear out the batteries to silence it, and flop back into bed again. If you behaved like this would you be surprised if you were burned in your bed?

Herbal medicine, properly used, aims to treat the *cause* of dis-ease in the body.

• THE ACTIVE PRINCIPLES OF HERBS •

What many people now seem to forget in their headlong pursuit of the countrified and natural is that herbs are in fact powerful chemical factories, which must be used with care. Herbs' nutritional and medical value comes from the presence of the many complex chemical substances in them which herbalists call their 'active principles'. The advantage that herbs have over man-made chemicals is that nature sensibly packages her chemicals in such well balanced and minute amounts that their safe assimilation by the body is assured. While chemical medicine is used solely to suppress disease, herbalists use nature's chemicals to stimulate the body's inherent healing power. By reaching right down to the cause, not the symptom, they ensure a gradual return to full recovery. Chemical medicine seems much more spectacular, superficially at least, because it produces such quick results. But by merely blocking out the symptoms it fails to achieve a real cure, and if the illness is chronic and needs prolonged treatment, the build-up of powerful chemicals in the system over a long period can reap some horrid dividends.

• SYNERGY •

I believe that plants are not simply the safest way to give medicine but are also the most effective not just because they can be easily assimilated (the green blood of the plant, its chlorophyll, is very similar in its molecular structure to the haemoglobin in our own blood), but because they are capable of working synergistically. This means that two or more herbs correctly mixed together result in a whole which is greater than the sum of its parts. This may sound a bit farfetched, but monitored companion planting has endorsed this. It seems that certain plants that are grown next to one another not only act as allies, fending off undesirable insects, but strengthen each other in all sorts of ways. For example, nettles have been proved to increase the volatile oil content of such plants as sage, valerian and angelica. Some herbs properly combined with others act to make the way in which their companion works better. An example is the griping action of senna pods which can be soothed by the addition of an aromatic herb, such as ginger. Some herbs combined with specific allies act in completely different ways on the body. For example, lobelia mixed with peppermint and made into a syrup with honey acts as an expectorant helping to ease mucus up from the lungs, but mix it with cascara and it will rapidly and smoothly clear the bowel.

• KIRLIAN PHOTOGRAPHY •

Another aspect of synergy is shown by the fact that chemical constituents in plants cannot be mimicked synthetically because no chemist has yet found a way of reproducing the energy field that is present in every living thing. In this way there is more to a herb than the sum of its parts. That such an energy field exists has been indisputably proven by Kirlian photography. That it makes a quantifiable contribution to someone's health is harder to prove, though there is an expanding body of research being conducted into just this proposition. Kirlian photography is one of the physical proofs of what herbalists call the presence of a healing force. A Russian engineer Semyon Kirlian and his wife, while experimenting in the 1950s, found that high frequency pictures could distinguish between dead and living objects. Dead ones had a thin and constant outline, living ones were subject to changes. The living objects' activity was also visible in a great variety of colour patterns and the Russians, one of the few peoples to take this discovery seriously, are now using Kirlian photography to diagnose diseases which can't be discovered by any other means. They believe that in most illnesses there is a pre-clinical phase where physical symptoms have not yet manifested and they say it is possible to predict a disease by photographing this phase. Kirlian photography can also tell us much about plants. The electromagnetic field round a raw vegetable is very bright and extended compared to that round the same vegetable when cooked.

• HARVESTING •

To my mind there is a subtle but indispensable difference between the chemical compounds extracted from plants and the chemical structure created synthetically in the laboratory and herbalists have always had a profound respect for this difference. Culpeper's instruction to harvest a herb on 'the south side of the hill, with a clear heart just before the summer sun touches the mid-point' is neither arcane nor superstitious. Any herb facing south gets more sun, which will ensure a greater potency and concentration of its essential oils and resins. If that herb is picked at the height of a warm summer's day it will be perfectly dry and so will not rot with mildew in the course of its subsequent processing. A clear heart is also important – recent studies in immunology have shown that negative emotions alter both our internal and external chemistry. Sweaty hands can be produced by negative emotions and will result in acidity which will in turn alter the chemical constituents of a plant if such acid sweat gets onto it. One also needs careful concentration and smooth action when harvesting plants. Jerking and tearing them inevitably destroys some of their valuable healing properties. Herbalists were once forbidden to harvest herbs with anything made of iron as it was thought to damage the plants' energy. For this reason I store my herbs in glass rather than plastic and never use copper or aluminium vessels to prepare them.

• VITAL FORCE •

The concept of energy goes even further. Herbalists believe there is a vital energy inside every human being which science is unable to quantify and which they call the 'vital force'. It is an internal intelligence which is chiefly concerned with maintaining the body's equilibrium, a process modern science calls homoeostasis. If this delicate balance, this homoeostasis, can be encouraged, the whole person will enjoy good health. If it is disturbed the result is disease.

A good herbalist is concerned not merely with the symptom of a disease but more importantly with finding out why the body has not been able to heal itself. Even orthodox medicine acknowledges that an astonishing number of ailments are self-limiting. Herbalists try to direct the vital force by encouraging it with herbal treatments which stimulate the body's own defences to produce the desired return to positive health. The remedies they use are individually tailored to the patient's needs, so that two patients with the same disease may be treated with quite different prescriptions, simply because the underlying causes of the disease might be quite different in each individual.

• HOW HERBAL REMEDIES WORK •

Patients cannot be standardised, nor can their medicines, if they are to be truly effective. This fact presents the pharmaceutical industry with an enormous problem, because it must produce drugs in huge quantities, whilst the recipients of such drugs remain, thank goodness, stubbornly individual. This is another reason why there is such wide spread disillusionment with modern drug therapy. One woman's aspirin can be another woman's stomach ulcer.

Herbal remedies work in many different ways. Some work partly through their mucilaginous components; marshmallow root and comfrey root are particularly rich in mucilage which soothes and provides physical protection and relief from irritation and pain externally and internally. Tannins and other chemicals contained in plants such as witch hazel and bistort form tough antiseptic coats over exposed tissue or mucous membrane. Senna works by gently irritating the bowels to produce elimination. Powerful herbs like chilli, garlic and ginger stimulate the blood vessels to increase the flow of blood through the tissues, and bitter herbs like gentian stimulate the range of digestive reflexes. Some herbs act as expectorants, for example mullein and lobelia, causing you to cough up mucus and others act as diuretics on the urinary system. All these responses act to protect the body in some way.

Herbal remedies are also capable of adjusting bodily processes. They do this by acting almost like foods rather than medicines. For example, a herbal tincture extracted from oat straw can relieve nervous exhaustion; this is as a result of its rich mineral and nutrient content as well as the dynamic action of constituent chemicals. Some remedies are capable of increasing blood flow and yet slowing the heart rate, thereby nurturing a heart under strain; an example is hawthorn. Ginseng acts as an adaptogen, this means it enables all other herbs and foods taken into the body to work more effectively. It also acts specifically to improve the ability of the adrenal cortex to respond to stress - the adrenal medulla is where the hormone adrenalin is manufactured.

Herbal remedies are superb at helping to eliminate toxins from the system. They are particularly good at improving the action of the bowels, kidneys, lungs, lymphatic system and liver all of which are involved in eliminating toxins from the body. They will work both on the body in general and on specific organs, helping to nourish and drain them. Herbalists are famous for being able to clean out the body to a degree that other therapists cannot match.

• EMPIRICAL TESTING •

The one thing that is outstandingly in favor of herbal medicine is that it has been empirically tested for thousands of years on those inimitable non-standard laboratory animals, human beings. I believe this empirical testing is far more important than any double-blind crossover trial. I think the millions of dollars spent on such trials are of doubtful value, otherwise why would such horrors as thalidomide have been unleashed on the market? The reason I think such trials are unimportant is that human beings remain stubbornly individual. How can controlled conditions and reproducible results apply in a non-standardisable unique person? Besides all this, the double-blind clinical trial approach is a fail-ure as far as nutrients such as essential fatty acids are concerned. It cannot cope with highly complex substances with a host of potent metabolites and nutritional cofactors on which bodily activity depends.

WHO stated in 1978 that 'Traditional medicine has a holistic approach, i.e. that of viewing man in his totality within a wide ecological spectrum, and of emphasising that ill health or disease is bought about by an imbalance, or disequilibrium, of man in his total ecological system and not only by the causative agent and pathogenic evolution.'

Hippocrates, often deemed to be the father of medicine, acknowledged all these components thousands of years ago. He knew that what a person does, thinks or says, what they eat and drink, the conditions in which they live and what they work at, were not simply the reasons for their illness but *often the only conditions that needed treatment.*

• BACH FLOWER REMEDIES •

It is also possible to treat the mind, the spirit or the emotions with herbal remedies. Edward Bach was a famous exponent of this approach. A most unusual healer, he died in 1936 aged 50, having devised a system known as the Bach Flower Remedies. He believed that warmed dew absorbed the properties of the plant from whose surface it was collected. The collection of dew was a tedious and difficult task but he had the idea of putting flowers in a glass bowl full of pure spring water and leaving them to stand in full sunlight for a few hours. This was a very effective way of impregnating the water with the power of the plant. He then bottled the water in dark glass bottles, preserving it with some brandy. Out of this stock bottle he took a few drops and added them to one ounce of pure spring water. The patient was instructed to take four drops of this diluted remedy in a little water four times a day. He believed that these floral remedies could correct the disharmonies of personality and emotion. 'The main reason for the failure of modern medicine,' he wrote in 1931, 'is that it is dealing with results not causes. Diseases are in essence the result of conflict between soul and mind . . . the mind being the most delicate and sensitive part of the body shows the onset and cause of the disease much more definitely than the body. The individual is treated and as he becomes well the disease goes.' Although his ideas related to the highest orders of consciousness there is nothing particularly complicated or esoteric about the remedies. He intended them to be for simple home use and anybody can be their own Bach flower practitioner. Bach Flower remedies deal with a wide range of emotions from loneliness, fear and uncertainty, through to despondency, grief, anger, guilt or shock. From my own experience I can say they work brilliantly. Nor do they work simply as a result of some sort of clever psychotherapy. I have added them to other remedies without telling the recipient that I have even given them a Bach flower remedy and seen the most marvellous ease and transformation take place.

• HERBS: BEWARE •

Having said all this I should point out that not all herbs are kind and harmless. Herbal medicine, properly administered, is gentle and heals slowly at a deep rooted level (as a rough yard stick I tell my patients to allow one month of treatment for every year they have been ill) but there are some vicious and extremely poisonous herbs around. Nature is not entirely beneficent, gentle and forgiving. An overdose of *Iris versicolour*, blue flag, will not merely stimulate the liver but will induce nausea, vomiting and colic. Socrates was given a dose of hemlock as his death potion. So powerful are the paroxysms it causes that it was mixed with opium poppy (*Papaver somniferum*) to allay the spasms. In large doses the milky white sap from the opium poppy's calyx can induce death, in lesser doses merely sleep and pain relief; yet let the seeds mature for only four or five more days and they can be safely baked in a nutritious poppy seed cake.

CHAPTER 2:

DIET, THE BEDROCK OF ALL GOOD HEALTH

The reasons for poor health are at least threefold. Firstly there are the obvious physical causes such as an insect sting, a sports injury, a burn or food poisoning. Secondly there are the circumstances in which we live, including damp or noisy housing, exposure to high levels of radiation and other pollutants and poor working conditions such as sub-standard lighting and seating, which will result in postural misalignment. Thirdly, and in my view probably the most important of all, is the emotional component. Grief, shock, anger, frustration and other negative emotions can be just as potent a cause of disease as any physical factor.

So by launching into the reasons why eating properly is the indispensable foundation of all good health I am *not* implying that nothing else matters. We need clean air and sunshine as well as the plants on which we are so dependent. In common with all other animals we need regular exercise and because our minds are indelibly linked to our bodies we also have deep spiritual and psychological needs. If these are not all adequately met, eventually our bodies will show the symptoms of dis-ease.

• STARVING TO DEATH •

By nature I'm optimistic but even I can see that the poor are getting poorer and growing poverty means increased malnutrition. Nearly twenty-five per cent of countries in the developing world are starving – the highest percentage in human history – while obesity has become an epidemic in the West.

Obesity is certainly a different kind of malnutrition, but nevertheless it is malnutrition, a peculiar form of starvation induced by ingesting empty calories, that is, food with no nutritional value at all. In January 1983 the Royal College of Physicians of London confirmed that, in common with people in the USA and other Western countries, the British, particularly the young, are getting fatter even though they are actually eating less than their ancestors were fifty years ago. Sixty per cent of all American children are obese and ninety per cent could not pass a rudimentary physical fitness test such as doing one push-up. By the time Californian girls are nine, eighty per cent have already been on their first diet! The burning question is not so much the quantity but the *quality* of the food we eat.

What we eat can literally kill or cure us. Hippocrates' ancient axiom 'let food be your medicine and medicine your food' has been endorsed by the WHO. All major medical and governmental agencies now agree that solving problems which arise from dietary mistakes would reduce the instances of diseases such as cancer. Eighty per cent of all cancers are now acknowledged to be at least partially induced by incorrect nutrition. The same is true of cardiovascular disease and even notoriously conservative bodies like the British Medical Association (BMA) are beginning to worry that this might also be true of chronic degenerative diseases.

Poor quality food is incapable of making good body chemistry and the average Western refined diet is so poor that it cannot hope to supply us with all we need for positive glowing health. Real food is rapidly disappearing. Almost ninety-eight per cent of everything we eat passes through the hands, or more accurately the machines, of food processors. Yet in the UK there is only one qualified nutritionist to approximately every seventeen food companies.

• CHEMICAL FOOD •

The problem is not so much what is taken out of our food, but what is added. Chemicals such as flavour stabilisers, enhancers, emulsifiers, acidulants, plasticisers, colours, extenders, preservatives, and stabilisers rank high on the list. More than *one billion* pounds of chemicals are added to food in the USA every year. Britain allows more additives and has weaker controls on them than any other major industrialised country. Not many additives have been tested for safety simply because of the enormous numbers involved; those that have were tested in the so-called scientific double-blind trial manner, in other words one at a time, on healthy well-fed animals. Out there in the real world we are much more likely to be eating lots of different additives all at once and their composition could be further altered by differing methods of cooking. By the age of twelve most of us have eaten a half pound of coal-tar dyes, and as adults we eat five pounds of additives every year. Many of us are intensely susceptible to them. In 1984 Dr John Hunter, a specialist in food allergy with extensive experience dealing with migraine, asthma, rhinitis, urticaria, eczema, Crohn's disease and other digestive disorders, stated that one-fifth of his patients reacted to food additives.

It seems food technology rules and technological food simply can't be made without dozens of chemicals. A few enlightened supermarkets are heading the growing groundswell of public opinion against additives and are actively removing all unnecessary ingredients and contentious food additives which are believed to cause unpleasant reactions, but the snack market whose labels read like a chemistry set is growing by ten per cent a year.

Do yourself a favour: if the label on a product reads anything even slightly like something from a chemistry set, don't buy it. The small print on the label of many convenience foods admitting to a 'permitted colouring' or 'permitted antioxidant' covers a multitude of sins. Take the latter by way of example: two of the antioxidants which are widely used to prevent fats and oils from going rancid, butylated hydroxyanisole (BHA) and butylated hydroxytoluene (BHT), are cumulative. That is, they are easily stored in body fat if eaten in substantial amounts, and they are present in virtually all manufactured foods containing any form of fat. BHA has been proved to upset the proper functioning of the intestinal muscles. BHT is believed to increase levels of fat and cholesterol in the blood, to induce birth abnormalities, stunted growth and baldness, liver and kidney damage and noticeable changes in brain chemistry. The UK Standards Committee has twice recommended that neither antioxidant be used in food, yet it is still widely used in many of the convenience foods which contain fat.

• LIVING FOOD •

How can you hope to build healthy living cells on dead, chemicalised, processed foods? Dr Max Bircher-Benner, a Swiss nutritionist and a visionary before his time, understood this very well. 'Mangez-vivant!', he would say to his patients, meaning 'eat living food'. He had no objections to eating meat as long at it was uncooked and in its entirety of blood, fat, bones, entrails, skin and flesh. In other words, the way a lion eats prey in the wild. And how many of us would be willing to do that? He maintained that as soon as anything was processed in some way it altered the state of the whole food energy and produced ill health. Later experiments with cats provided evidence for this view. Cats fed on a raw diet flourished over several generations while those fed on cooked meat developed all sorts of malformaties and health problems including allergies, and genetic problems. Dr Bircher-Benner maintained that while nutrition may not be 'the highest thing in life . . . it is the soil on which the highest things can either perish or flourish'.

• SOIL AND CHEMICAL FERTILISERS •

Healthy soil is one of the World's greatest natural resources and this rich, nutrient – packed layer of the Earth's crust from which food crops draw their sustenance is currently being lost at the rate of twenty-four billion tonnes a year. This is the result of intensive farming with large amounts of chemical fertilisers, coupled with monoculture and the ploughing up of margin lands. This is undoubtedly a global crisis because, as an article in *New Scientist* pointed out, what is at stake is not only the degradation of soil, but the degradation of life itself.

One thousand million gallons of liquid pesticide are now being used yearly on Britain's farms. The London Food Commission's report 'Food Adulteration and How to Beat it' states that of the 426 main chemicals legally used in 3,009 brands of pesticides and fertilisers, 164 have been implicated in causing cancer, genetic mutations, irritant reactions and reproductive problems ranging from impotence to birth defects. The record for the number of times a single lettuce has been sprayed according to Friends of the Earth is forty-six, onions fifteen and potatoes eight. My advice? Eat organically as far as you can and if you can't find organic food write to organisations that can help you. Thump the counter of every shop and supermarket you go into demanding organic foods. Safeway's supplies of organically grown food quickly disappear off the shelves in spite of higher prices. Such enthusiasm speaks volumes for our growing concern about the contamination of our environment. If you simply can't find organic food wash all fruits really well and scrub vegetables in hot water. I soak mine, after giving them a good wash, in a basin full of cold water with half a cup of apple cider vinegar added. Full of potassium, the vinegar helps to restore the alkaline balance of the skins. There is also a natural pesticide remover on the market based on aloe vera (see Resource Directory).

• SUGAR •

I recently phoned a friend who is a food chemist and asked what he thought was added to processed food the most. His reply? Sugar. He said it goes with almost everything and masquerades under all sorts of labels. Sucrose, glucose, dextrose, various syrups, fructose, lactose, honey, invert sugar (rather like synthetic honey), maple syrup, molasses, treacle, Sorbitol, Mannitol, Xylitol. Of the hundred pounds of sugar we eat on average each year, *seventy pounds are hidden in processed foods.* Sugars are preservatives, bulking agents, cheap sweeteners and give what food technologists call 'mouth-feel'.

You might expect to find sugar in soft drinks, but it is also present in some brands of frozen peas and the manufactured muesli which so many people eat, imagining it to be a health food'. And have you ever thought how much sugar there is in an average-sized bottle of Coke? One tablespoon! More than enough to depress the ability your white blood cells have to engulf and destroy bacteria for hours. Certainly enough to begin the long slide downhill to tooth decay. The fact is we don't need any sugar. It contains no additional nutrients. Even unbleached sugar is simply unwashed white sugar and contains only traces of some minerals which are more abundantly available from other sources. It is full only of "empty" calories. The ubiquitous drink also contains acidifying agents, salts and buffering agents, emulsifiers, carriers like ethyl alcohol, foaming or antifoaming agents, synthetic vitamin C, caffeine and, of course, chemical preservatives.

If you need to sweeten anything use date sugar, made from dried and ground dates, maple syrup or organic honey, and be sparing with it. There is growing evidence that these and indeed all other sugars suppress the function of the immune system and are increasingly implicated in emotional disorders ranging from anxiety and depression to schizophrenia.

• SALT •

We eat far too much salt. Certainly in its natural form it keeps the body fluids in balance, but it is almost **never** nutritionally essential to add salt to food. Talking salt with food is an acquired not an inborn taste. The only circumstances in which it is necessary to add salt to your diet is when you do long strenuous exercise in extremely hot weather to which you have not had a chance to acclimatise.

Ninety per cent of the salt you eat is actually hidden in food. The amount of salt needed daily by an adult in a temperate climate is four grams and this can always be obtained from natural food. Most people add so much salt to their diet that their intake can be as much as 20 grams a day. Canned and processed foods invariably have added salt, and the additives in them, including monosodium glutamate, sodium bicarbonate, sodium nitrite, sodium benzoate, sodium propionate and sodium citrate, also contain salt. Some foods which contain salt may surprise you, for example, hard cheeses, dried, evaporated or condensed milk, baking powder and breakfast cereals. It is important to realise that all salt, whether it be rock or plain table salt, has virtually the same chemical composition and sodium content; so there is no point in just switching to another kind because it sounds healthier.

The more salt you ingest the more calcium you secrete. If you sprinkle anything with salt before cooking it draws both the minerals and the natural juices out of it. It is also interesting to note that in artificially fertilised foods the sodium content is higher and the potassium content lower whereas in organic foods the reverse is the case. Sodium and potassium are mutually antagonistic. The correct potassium/sodium balance should be 80:20 and when this is disturbed the body quickly fills up with toxins because the pressure between different body fluids is disturbed. Symptoms include swelling, chronic lassitude and poor immunity.

My advice, therefore, is to cut all forms of salt out of your diet completely and remember that processed foods are too high in sodium and too low in potassium. There is, for example, one hundred times more sodium in canned vegetable soup than in a fresh home-made one. Unsalted food initially tastes strange but be generous with your herbs and spices and soon you will notice salted food tastes terrible and leaves you feeling thirsty. Not only does a salt-free diet reduce high blood pressure and the possibility of strokes, but for slimmers on a typical high-fat diet the pounds and inches really begin to shrink when you cut out all forms of salt. While weaning yourself off salt try this variation on Japanese gomosio.

A variation on Japanese gomosio

- Stir 8oz of sesame meal constantly in a heavy-bottomed frying pan until heated through and toasted.

- Decant and add it to 1 oz of powdered vegetable bouillon (see Resources Directory) and mix well.

- Decant and cool. Store in a covered container.

- Alternatively, if you want something with even more zip, mix two parts of kelp powder with one part of dried parsley, one of dried marjoram, one of garlic powder and one of cayenne pepper. Use this to flavour your meals as you once used salt.

• ALKALISING YOUR SYSTEM •

This excellent recipe will not only alkalise your system – eating too much meat, fish, eggs, dairy products, alcohol, salt, sugar and caffeine makes your body acid – but will also help to correct your sodium/potassium ratios and detoxify your system. Potassium broth is particularly helpful if taken during a fast. This makes a great-tasting addition to any cleansing programme and will flush your system of unwanted salts and acids while giving you a concentrated amount of vitamins and minerals.

Potassium Broth

It is important to use organic vegetables to make Potassium Broth. You do not want to consume any toxic insecticides or chemical fertilisers while you are on a cleansing and detoxification programme.

Drink one pint or more daily, warmed. Store strained excess in the fridge for up to two days in a glass container and reheat as needed.

- Fill one-quarter of a large pot with thickly cut potato peelings, then add equal amounts of carrot peelings and whole chopped beetroot, chopped onions and garlic, and celery and greens. Add hot chilli peppers to taste.

- Add enough water to cover the vegetables and simmer on very low heat for one to two hours.

- Strain the liquid and drink only the broth. Put the vegetables on the compost.

- Make enough for two days; refrigerate left-over broth. Then start a fresh broth.

• FATS •

It has long been known that eating too much saturated fat causes all sorts of problems including plaquing of the arteries which can lead to heart disease, strokes and even cancer. A lot of fat is hidden in sausages, baked goods and dairy products, as well as salt and sugar.

- Saturated fat raises blood cholesterol and increases the risk of heart attacks. It is present in *all dairy products and animal flesh* but the only two vegetable sources of it are coconut and palm oil.
- Unsaturated fats (mono or polyunsaturated) are high in calories so will

help you get fat but have good effects on blood fats, because the more unsaturated fat in the bloodstream, the less room for saturated fats.
● Some of the more persistent residues from pesticides latch on to animal fats. A government survey found pesticide residues in one-third of all sausages sampled, half of 150 burgers sampled and half of 177 cheeses sampled.

BUTTER V. MARGARINE

Let me explain how margarine is made. The pure liquid polyunsaturated oil is hardened by pushing hydrogen gas through it, a process called *hydrogenation*; **a process which converts it to a totally saturated fat**. This is one of the greatest unexposed and poorly understood scandals in the history of the food manufacturing industry! Besides this, margarine is very close to plastic in its molecular structure and is an absolutely dead food. It will not support any type of bacteria or fungus, nor will it melt naturally when you roll it between your fingers. What do you think it does while it is inside your body? It will certainly give you the same number of calories as butter, the added bonus of betacarotene and annatto (additional colouring) and it often includes mono and diglycerides and maltodextrim and it could plaque up your arteries. A study by Harvard Medical School of 85,095 women, followed over eight years, found that those eating margarine had an *increased* risk of coronary heart disease.

The oils used in margarine are overly refined so their essential fatty acids (EFAs) are damaged. Insult is added to injury with further refinement, using solvents from petroleum to produce a lighter taste, clarity and colour. Bleach further removes EFAs, trace minerals and vitamins. Heat (as when frying) further damages the EFAs and the resulting oxidation creates damaging free radicals in the body, dramatically increasing your need for vitamins and minerals.

During the process of hydrogenation itself, trans fatty acids (TFAs) are produced which have a different molecular structure to anything found in human tissues. These have a negative effect on our body's ability to use EFAs.

The dangers of TFAs are complex but important; they appear to disrupt the body's use of cholesterol. Because our bodies can't process low density compounds which carry cholesterol the cells simply work harder to synthesise cholesterol, so raising levels of cholesterol in the blood.

There is a non-hydrogenated margarine just coming on to the market called Vitaquel. This is solidified with lecithin but it is often quite hard to come by. When buying margarine, look for the clear wording on the packing which says either not- or non-hydrogenated and make sure there is nothing chemical added. This type of margarine should not be used for cooking or frying. Avoid anything that has been hydrogenated. This includes not only many brands of margarine, but also almost all baked goods, canned sauces, cheese snacks, potato chips, including corn chips, and chocolate. Get your EFAs from walnuts, linseed (and their unheated oils), evening primrose oil, blackcurrant seed oil and beans and pulses.

OLIVE OIL

Olive oil actually **lowers** your cholesterol levels by reducing the low density lipoproteins (LDLs), which cause heart disease, and increasing high density lipoproteins (HDLs), which protect us from heart disease. But remember olive oil is still high in calories so use it sparingly and check it is cold pressed (unprocessed). Refined oils are treated with chemicals including caustic soda to remove fatty acids then bleached and deodorised by heating at high temperatures for up to twelve hours. Their chemical structure is so altered they have no health benefits.

Heating any oil up to smoking temperature, however it began (mono-, poly-, or saturated), again distorts its chemical structure and encourages the proliferation of free radicals in the body, so deep frying is not a good idea. When heating olive oil it is an excellent idea to put a little hot water in the bottom of the pan first. This will stop it from getting too hot.

SYNTHETIC FATS

Food manufacturers are falling over themselves to develop 'non-fat fats' and so grab a slice of the extremely profitable slimming market. Avoid them. Fluffed up with cellulose, synthetic sweeteners and additives, they are entirely artificial and unhealthy. Low-fat spreads are generally made of butter diluted by half with water and then further coloured or emulsified. So why not get some pure real butter and use it sparingly?

• DAIRY PRODUCTS •

The milk of any species was designed for one purpose only; to feed its young. Humans are the only creatures on earth who regularly drink the milk designed for another species as part of their normal diet.

The enzymes we need to break down and digest milk are rennin and lactose. By the age of four, many of us lose the ability to digest lactose because we can no longer synthesise the digestive enzyme lactase. This lactose intolerance results in diarrhoea, flatulence and stomach cramps. It has been suggested that some ninety per cent of adult Asian and black people, and twenty per cent of Caucasian children, are lactose intolerant.

COWS' MILK

To the list of problems naturally inherent in human consumption of milk designed for baby cows I can add a whole host of unnatural ones. Cows' milk contains the accumulated pesticides that have been sprayed on the grain fed to cattle, and the female hormones given to cows to increase milk production and body fat. The newly proposed use of the hormone Bovine Somatotropin (BST) in milk may change its chemical composition and presents an uncertain and as yet unchartered danger to humans. Some milk has been shown to contain trace metals and radioactivity at higher levels than those permissible in drinking water. Some twenty per cent of milk-producing cows in America are infected with leukaemia viruses which, because milk is pooled when collected, infects the whole milk supply. These cancer-inducing viruses are resistant to being killed by pasteurisation and have been recovered from supermarket supplies. Can it be a coincidence that the highest rates of leukaemia are found in children aged three to thirteen who consume the most milk products, and dairy farmers who, as a profession, have the highest rate of leukaemia of any occupational group?

ALTERNATIVES

However, there is some good news. There are many delicious and healthy alternatives to milk and dairy products. My favourite are soya products. Almost everything that you can get as a dairy product is available in its soya form including ice-cream, cream, milk, cheese and butter. Some of these are even beginning to appear in supermarkets and all of them are available in health food shops. There are also some excellent soya yogurts available sweetened with apple juice; it is possible to make your own soya yogurt. Rice milk can be found in some health food shops.

Nut milks are a delicious alternative to dairy milk and are easily made at home.

Almond Milk

- Half a cup of almonds. Four cups of water. Honey to taste.

- Blend in a liquidiser and strain.

- For a whiter, blander milk, skin the almonds first by soaking them in boiling water, draining and pinching the fat end of each almond between the thumb and forefinger. The nut will simply slide out.

• EGGS •

Eggs are fibreless and are very high in fat and cholesterol. In fact, they contain eight times more cholesterol than the equivalent weight of beef. They are also regularly implicated in cases of salmonella food poisoning. Indeed one of Britain's leading microbiologists has advised that people over 65 years of age, anyone who is ill, pregnant women and babies, should avoid eggs altogether except in baking.

There are some interesting things about eggs that you may not know. Somewhere between one and five colourants are fed to chickens to give a richer colouring to egg yolks. One of these, canthaxanthin, was actually banned by the British Ministry of

Agriculture, Food and Fishery (MAFF), for direct human consumption. I wonder what it is doing in animal feed? Chickens are also fed arsenic to kill parasites and stimulate growth, and naturally some of this ends up in their eggs.

If you must eat eggs, at least ensure that the ones you choose are free range, as the average battery chicken is bred in horrific conditions. Battery chickens have their beaks trimmed and their forward vision restricted because they become vicious in such appalling caged conditions. By nature, they do not peck at each other if bred on the open range. Having said this, you should know that free range chickens still have their beaks trimmed.

I have found soya cream is an excellent substitute for eggs in baking. Use one level tablespoonful in place of an egg.

• MEAT •

Before I start this section I must declare my convictions and allegiance. I am a committed vegan. Initially I became one simply on the grounds of health. When I began my research into this subject I discovered that countries in which the most red meat was consumed suffer proportionately the highest rate of death from heart attacks, strokes, cancer and diabetes.

RED MEAT AND DISEASE

The most prevalent kind of cancer in men and women in the Western world is colon rectal cancer, which accounts for sixty per cent of all cancers. Red meat is heavily implicated in colon rectal cancer. The probable reason for this is that when the cholesterol in meat is digested, by-products are created which are powerful carcinogens. For example, when beef is barbecued the fat that splatters into the fire is changed by the heat into benzopyrene, a potent carcinogen. This chemical rises in the smoke, coating the surface of the steak and when the meat is chewed and swallowed it is smeared against the bowel wall during the course of the digestive process.

Just as importantly for women, a diet high in red meat increases the risk of cancer of the breast. This is because cows, lambs and pigs bred for slaughter are fed hormones and antibiotics, the residues of which remain in active form in the meat. Women who eat animal fat create high levels of the hormones oestrogen and prolactin, and these both stimulate the growth of breast tissue, the lining of the uterus and many other tissues. As a result they have higher rates of tumours and cancers of both the breast and uterus.

All forms of concentrated protein, including chicken, fish and eggs, as well as meat, injure the kidney filters contributing to kidney failure, as well as leaching calcium from the bones, leading to osteoporosis.

Meat also contributes to chronic inflammatory conditions, whether they be of the bronchial tubes or joints. This may be the result of over stimulation of the immune system from constant assault by foreign animal products which are inherent in all meat and dairy products. It seems that fragments of animal proteins wend their way into the circulatory system after meals containing these substances. Anti-bodies which work against the protein in milk as well as against beef muscle are commonly found in the blood of carnivores. A few years ago the Lancet reported that animal protein and animal fat actually aggravated arthritis symptoms, and every single one of those patients put on a pure vegan diet noticed a significant improvement very quickly. Ninety per cent of asthmatics placed on a vegan diet were able to reduce, and some were even able to discontinue entirely, their medications. I could fill half this book with the mounting evidence that has been accumulating over the last ten years that a high-fibre, low-fat plant-based diet is of central importance in both the prevention and treatment of an incredibly broad range of diseases. It has been estimated that vegans account for only forty per cent of the national cancer rate and increase their life span by a minimum of six years.

ALTERNATIVES

The alternatives to red meat are many and varied, and apart from preparing vegetables and pulses in interesting and different ways, you can experiment with tofu, tempeh, texturised vegetable protein (TVP), Quorn and Quinoa.

Remember, it's not what you do five per cent of the time that matters. I've been known to indulge in champagne and Belgian chocolates. It's what you do ninety-five per cent of the time to build and maintain health that really matters.

It took me six years to move entirely over to veganism so if you do take the plunge do it at a pace that feels comfortable to you. The only time I would suggest a quick change is if somebody has a potentially life-threatening disease, in which case they need to decide to embrace veganism as soon as possible. Long years of clinical experience have convinced me that veganism is the fastest way I can accelerate a patient to health, coupled with periods of fasting and raw food. Fish was the last thing I cut from my diet. Looking back, years later, when I review the evidence of how we treat our rivers and seas, I often wonder why. We use them like large open sewers pouring millions of gallons of faeces, urine, discarded drugs, sanitary towels and other horrific ingredients into our costal waters **daily.** Poor fish!

● FISH ●

POLLUTION

When I tell people I am a vegan they often assume that although I don't eat meat and dairy products, I will eat fish. Indeed fish and fish oils are often described as particularly helpful to a healthy diet, but consider this. Rivers and oceans are often heavily contaminated with pesticides and toxic chemical residues, so much so it is almost impossible nowadays to find fish from unpolluted waters. Bigger fish often eat little fish and as a result of this progression the larger fish can have dangerously high concentrations of pesticides, insecticides and other toxic chemicals in their bodies. All fish are exposed to detergents, industrial effluents, oil spillage, harbour dredgings, human and animal sewage, and ships' garbage. In view of all this, unsurprisingly, fish have been found to contain toxins known to be carcinogenic, and to cause kidney failure, nerve damage and birth defects. The fish themselves, swimming as they are in waters laced with carcinogenic chemicals, display alarmingly high rates of cancer. Pollutants like polychlorinated biphenyls (PCBs), DDT and Dioxin concentrate in the muscle tissue of fish and it has been estimated that eating a one pound fish from Lake Ontario is the same as drinking 1.5 million quarts of that polluted water. More than eighty per cent of the fish taken from lakes and rivers in New York State, Ohio and Michigan, showed cancerous tumours of the skin and liver visible to the eye. Carcinogenic hydro carbons were found in fish in rivers in Maryland, in the Nile, and in rivers in Florida, and there are increasingly alarming reports of carcinogenic residues in fish taken from the Mediterranean and Baltic seas.

SHELLFISH

These pollutants particularly affect creatures like carp which live at the bottom of the ocean, river or lake where the chemicals fall and concentrate. Oysters, clams and mussels have all been found with excessive levels of pollutants and, as filter feeders, they eliminate contaminants through their faecal matter. As humans usually prefer to eat clams and oysters whole they munch not only the toxins concentrated in the tissue but also trapped faecal matter left in the intestinal tract. In 1984 mussels in California were found to have lead contamination 150 times greater than the maximum said to be fit for human consumption. Shellfish are notorious carriers of toxic levels of lead, cadmium, arsenic and other heavy metals. Raw shellfish are renowned for carrying dangerous microbes and toxins and since the introduction of raw fish in increasingly popular Japanese restaurants in the Western world, infections from parasitic worms have increased.

MERCURY POISONING

Poisoning from mercury resulting in nerve paralysis, though still rare, is becoming increasingly common among fish eaters. Large predatory fish such as halibut, tuna, swordfish, shark and marlin are particularly predisposed to contamination by mercury. Mutagenic PCBs tend to gravitate to the flesh of trout, catfish, bass, carp, bluefish and mackerel, and mackerel are particularly fond of feeding off human sewage. The Irish Sea is the most radioactive sea in the world; contamination from nuclear power plants also affects fish.

• FISH OILS •

Over the last few years fish oils have been praised as specially protective against clogged arteries and heart disease. Think about this. The liver of the fish, like the liver of any human, is the central organ for processing chemicals, so the chemicals which accumulate in the flesh of the fish are particularly concentrated in its liver and *it is the liver of fish from which oil is extracted*. Fish oils that are described as providing protection to the arteries actually decrease the blood's ability to coagulate to stop bleeding. While the rate of heart attacks among Eskimos, who eat tons of fish, is very low, they suffer from the world's highest rate of cerebral haemorrhagic strokes, nose bleeds and epilepsy. Eskimos also have the highest osteoporosis rate in the world.

Fish oils have recently been found to increase the length of a normal pregnancy, and an overly long pregnancy will increase a baby's weight thus increasing the risk of birth accidents and the necessity for caesareans and even, in extreme cases, maternal deaths. Birth rates in the Faroe Islands are among the highest in the World and death rates in late pregnancy are alarmingly high, although the number involved are very low. Besides all this fish oil, like any other oil, except olive oil, contributes to gall-bladder disease and is high in cholesterol. Far from being brain food a lot of fish is so high in mercury that it actually poisons the brain and nerve cells!

• FARMED FISH •

The flesh of farmed salmon is made to look appetisingly pink by a dye mixed in with fish food. Farmed fish are kept in cages, so they breed diseases, just like broiler chickens; trout are particularly prone to this. Allegedly pesticides and antibiotics are regularly used by fish farms and allegedly, some fish farmers use Dichlorvos to get rid of sea lice in salmon. The US Environmental Protection Agency has classified this pesticide as a potential carcinogen and it is listed by the British Government as being one of the most dangerous chemicals that can enter our waterways. Yet until 1992 the British government was still condoning its use. Both the Dutch and German governments have warned their populace not to eat flat fish caught in the North Sea because they consider them too diseased with, amongst other things, liver disease, skin lesions, viral diseases and genetic abnormalities. North Sea fish are exposed to all sorts of environmental contaminants. So if you want to eat fish:

- buy from deeper, cleaner, oceans than the North Sea. Ask your fishmonger where it came from;
- cook it well;
- treat your own catch cautiously. Consider getting its purity confirmed by your local environmental health officer;
- don't buy frozen fish whose origins are not labelled or mixtures of fish in pre-prepared food such as fishfingers;
- campaign for cleaner waterways and seas. However, when doing this don't be disappointed when you hit blank walls. When Friends of the Earth asked for information about the quantity and toxicity of sewage sludge

supplied to farmers, their request was turned down by the local Water Authority who said; 'The names of individual farmers, their addresses, grid references of private farm land, etc., form part of the Register, but are clearly data of a personal nature we could not provide to others.'

The good news after all this gloom is that by significantly reducing your consumption of all meats, fish, dairy products and eggs, you will have an even lower risk of suffering from heart disease than the famous Eskimos, and a much lower risk of contracting osteoporosis.

I haven't mentioned the compassion side of the argument against all flesh food, and have chosen instead to concentrate purely on its health aspects, but let me say this. The Former Archbishop of Canterbury, Dr Robert Runcie, wrote the following about intensive livestock rearing: 'Of course the systems of extreme confinement are to be abhorred . . . History has repeatedly shown that when man exploits his fellow creatures for immediate gain, it rebounds on him eventually and leads to spiritual poverty.'

• DIET AND DISEASE •

No one diet suits every single person. Our nutritional needs are as different and as individual as our fingerprints. Literally, one woman's peanut can be another's poison.

It is now acknowledged that people's nutritional needs vary according to their lifestyle and stage of life and are certainly affected by such factors as stress, illness, puberty, pregnancy and lactation, the menopause and old age. But what is less clearly understood is that structural and enzymatic differences, partially caused by genetics, determine how an individual will absorb any nutrients. You may be continually urinating a nutrient away simply because your renal threshold for it is very low, or you may have insufficient intestinal bacteria to ensure the absorption or manufacture of a certain nutrient. Or, what a noted biochemist calls 'one of the fundamental wisdoms of the body . . . the wisdom to eat' may be impaired by any one of myriad reasons so that you cannot choose food wisely.

So with the best will in the world, and given the finest organic diet you can muster, I still recommend nature's superfoods to supplement your diet.

• THE VITAMIN AND MINERAL CONTROVERSY •

Very few vitamin and mineral supplements are derived from food. When you investigate them closely you sometimes find horrifying ingredients. If you were labouring under the illusion that manufacturers are grinding up fresh raw vegetables and organic fruits and grains, jettison that idea! Commercial vitamins and minerals are nearly always synthesised by the big pharmaceutical companies from exactly the same materials as drugs, coal-tar derivatives, petroleum products, animal by-products which include parts of their bodies and their faecal matter, pulverised rocks, stones, shells and metals. The United States Pharmacopoeia simply says that if a product looks similar under a microscope or any other form of laboratory analysis it is the same product regardless of what it is made from. For example, salicylic acid is considered identical whether it comes from wintergreen leaves or from boiling coal in carbolic and sulphuric acid. It also contains glycerin which may be made from fresh vegetable sources or boiled down animal carcasses, particularly the cartilage and hooves.

● SYNTHESISING SYNTHETIC VITAMINS AND MINERALS ●

Vitamins and minerals naturally present in food are bound to food complexes with carbohydrates, proteins and lipids, and the human body recognises only this entire food complex as food. Nearly all supplements are synthetic combinations of isolated vitamins and minerals which are not bound to anything and may have an entirely different chemical structure from those found in food. They are also formulated so they can boast of one hundred per cent of the daily recommended allowance on labels.

These synthetic formulae often ignore antagonistic and synergistic affects among vitamins and minerals, both as far as absorption and metabolic reactions are concerned. The chelating agent in wholefoods that assists absorption may be missing and synthetic calcium and iron are not well absorbed by humans. The process of chelating is chemically constructing a formulation so that it can be forced into the body's tissues. For example, monosodium glutamate forces the taste buds on the tongue wider open than they would normally go, in order to make something taste more of what it would normally taste of. So, tomatoes taste more tomatoey.

Mega doses of vitamin and mineral supplements are largely excreted simply because the uptake mechanism in the intestines cannot cope with them, which is why B-complex will turn urine yellow and make it smell strongly, and iron will blacken the faeces. Mega dosing is not simply a waste of money; it can also be dangerous. If the body relies on formulated supplements it is possible that it may get lazy or 'forget' how to extract the nutrients from food efficiently. In other words, mega doses may actually block the body's normal and natural wisdom. Bear in mind also that the clever technology which bought us chemical chelators, transporters and time release agents in an attempt to get round this problem, are in themselves synthetic. Such concentrates may affect sensitive people.

So I believe that it is better to get nutrients from natural sources because our bodies are designed to absorb nutrients from food. It isn't just how much you take of a nutritional supplement that matters, it is how much you *absorb*.

Most people are unaware that many preparations of Vitamin B12, Cyanocobalamin, are made from ground up cows' livers or activated sewage sludge. These cows' livers are overloaded already with steroids and antibiotics and the pesticides that cows ingest while eating. I will readily admit that faecal matter is natural but do you really want to eat it? Vitamin A is made from fish livers and I have already clearly outlined the toxic overload from these (see page 21). Vitamin D is made from radiated oil, Vitamin C from acid blends which can irritate the lining of sensitive digestive tracts and most minerals are simply made from pulverised and powdered shells and rocks. In today's environment where increasingly depressed immune systems are responsible for many serious illnesses, I can think of hundreds of reasons why all of these materials would be a health risk, not a benefit. Hence, my support of nature's Superfoods.

• THE SUPERFOODS •

SPIRULINA

This is one of the most concentrated, nutritious foods on earth. It is a blue/green algae which evolved 3 billion years ago and has nourished people in Central America and Africa for centuries. Because it has no hard cellulose in its cell walls, but is composed of soft mucopolysaccharides, its protein is beautifully digested and assimilated in the human body. Spirulina has the highest protein of any natural food (65 per cent or more), far more than animal and fish flesh (15–25 per cent), soybeans (35 per cent), eggs (12 per cent), or whole milk (3 per cent). And ninety-five per cent of this protein is digestible. This is particularly important for those suffering from intestinal malabsorption – coeliacs, those affected by candida, Crohn's disease, mucous colitis and many people over forty who have dwindling supplies of hydrochloric acid in their stomachs.

Life in the fat lane

Spirulina's fat content is only five per cent, far lower than almost any other protein source. Ten grams (one tablespoonful) has only thirty-six calories and virtually no cholesterol. So spirulina is a low-fat, low-calorie, cholesterol-free source of protein. In contrast, a large egg yields 300 mg of cholesterol and eighty calories but only has as much protein as one tablespoonful of spirulina.

Colon cleansing

Engevita nutritional yeast, chlorella and spirulina are the only forms of protein that are not mucoid forming in the intestines. Spirulina acts as a metabolic activator directly on the body's tissues at a cellular level, thus promoting increased activity which burns up mucus-forming substances, such as the wastes from meat, eggs and dairy products. It is an aggressive cleansing herb that empties toxins out of the body tissues into the lymph and is a superb addition in both fasting and colon-cleansing programmes.

Spirulina and Hypoglycaemia

The minimal amount of carbohydrate in spirulina, fifteen to twenty-five per cent, consists of two sugars which are easily absorbed by the body with minimum insulin intervention. Insulin is a hormone manufactured in the pancreas; it helps regulate blood sugar-levels. Spirulina supplies rapid energy without taxing the pancreas so it will not precipitate hypoglycaemia (low blood sugar level). Indeed, it is actively helpful for controlling the sweeping blood sugar curves which so debilitate hypoglycaemics; one more reason why it is so useful in a fast. It is also the richest source of B12 in food, higher than beef, liver, chlorella or sea vegetables, so it is highly recommended in a vegan diet. It actually reduces cholesterol, triglyceride and LDL levels. This may be partially due to its unusual and very high gamma linoleic acid (GLA) content. One tablespoonful of spirulina provides 100 mg of GLA, and dietary GLA helps heart conditions, PMS, obesity and arthritis.

Spirulina and Immunity

The unique colour in spirulina, phycocyanin, has been proved to stimulate the immune system and accelerate normal cell control functions to prevent the degeneration of malignancies or to inhibit their growth or reoccurrence. The National Cancer Institute in America has found the glycolipids in spirulina to be remarkably active against the AIDS virus.

Spirulina actually encourages the growth of helpful bacteria in the gut. Research has shown an increase in helpful lactobacillus bacteria over a hundred days. Spirulina has also been shown to increase the efficient absorption of Vitamin B1 inside the cecum, the murkiest part of the colon most prone to infestation by parasites, by forty-three per cent. Healthy lactobacillus helps better digestion and absorption of B1 protects from infection and stimulates the immune system.

Spirulina and Anaemia, Candida and Toxicity

The iron in spirulina is twice as absorbable as the iron found in vegetables and meat, therefore it is highly recommended for people prone to anaemia. Spirulina was used to treat the 160,000 children suffering from radiation poisoning at Chernobyl. Remember that we are all constantly exposed to background radiation from the atmosphere; leaking microwave ovens, electrical power lines, X-ray machines, illuminated neon signs, digital clock faces, garage door openers and flying. Spirulina also inhibits the growth of harmful bacteria, yeast and fungi, which is why it is important as part of a Candida controlling programme, and can heal internal bacterial infections. A diet of thirty per cent of spirulina has been shown to decrease the toxicity of inorganic mercury and other harmful chemicals radically, as well as antibiotics and anti-cancer drugs which can cause acute nephrotoxicity – poison of the kidneys.

CHLORELLA

This is another of the blue-green algaes and is second only to spirulina in its nutritional content. The cell wall of chlorella has to be artificially cracked to make the nutrients more available and increase their digestibility. For this reason, my first preference would always be for spirulina. Having said this, chlorella has some unique properties. Where spirulina is a multi-cell, spiral-shaped plant which grows in salty or brackish water, chlorella is a round, single-cell algae which grows in fresh water. It contains five times as much chlorophyll as spirulina. It is also different from spirulina because it contains Chlorella Growth Factor (CGF). In a classic study, fifty ten-year-old students given two grams of chlorella daily for 112 days outstripped their control group in height and weight over this period of time. Chlorella's capacity to stimulate growth in the young is probably due to its high content of RNA and DNA – nucleic acids – which are important building blocks for life. RNA and DNA accelerate growth in the young and help to repair damaged tissue in adults.

It has been suggested that the loss of energy and physical deterioration associated with ageing are due to the increasing breakdown of DNA and RNA which are needed to keep cells healthy. From around the age of twenty, our natural production of RNA and DNA becomes sluggish. A diet rich in DNA and RNA foods produces more energy and a more youthful appearance, and alleviates long-standing problems such as arthritis, memory loss and depression.

THE IMPORTANCE OF CHLOROPHYLL

All plant life depends upon the sun. We depend upon those plants. Sunlight activates the green chlorophyll in plants to generate energy for the plants. Molecules of chlorophyll are constructed around magnesium and carry oxygen around the inside of plant cells which in turn create energy for the plant. It is this stored energy in plants which we eat and absorb to sustain us. Plant energy is the primary energy of life because even carnivores eat animals which eat plants.

Our vitality depends upon a good supply of oxygen. Germs gravitate towards tissue which is oxygen deficient. Cancer tissues grow by a process which does not use oxygen.

The advantages of taking chlorophyll

Over the years I have noticed that those of my patients who tend to get viruses such as flus and colds are generally either anaemic or they are smokers. Fewer haemoglobin molecules mean reduced oxygen-carrying capacity for red blood cells. Smoking makes the haemoglobin of red blood cells bind with carbon monoxide, found in cigarette smoke. Whenever oxygen is wanting in our cells, disease sets in. Both chlorophyll and haemoglobin molecules are capable of carrying oxygen to cells and they are fairly similar in construction.

Many years of research have found that chlorophyll is not a chemical which is good for a specific disease but it benefits the entire body by carrying oxygen to every cell. Consequently chlorophyll can help many different conditions including sinusitis, colds, rhinitis, respiratory infections, colon problems including ulcerative colitis, high blood pressure, skin infections, pancreatitis, peptic ulcers, gastritis, mouth sores, boils, fatigue, cancer, septic wounds, and it increases resistance to X-rays.

Japanese researchers have found that the juice of any green plant inhibits chromosome damage which is one of the links in the chain of events leading to cancer.

All grasses contain fresh chlorophyll. There was a village in Austria during the Second World War which had all its food supplies commandeered by invading troops. The population was consequently forced to live off grass. Not only did the villagers thrive but many of their degenerative diseases began to heal completely. While you might blanch at the thought of eating grass, the good news is that other dark green vegetables such as spinach, cabbage and nettles also contain large amounts of chlorophyll as, of course, does chlorella.

The CGF factor noted in chlorella is also present in wheat and barley grass. To obtain all its benefits it must be administered orally or as a rectal injection and must be freshly made. Synthetic chlorophyll won't do and can be poisonous.

BARLEY AND WHEAT GRASSES

Barley and wheat grasses can be sprouted and the sprouts are more potent nutritionally than the grains themselves, being richly abundant with vitamins, minerals and chlorophyll. Barley is twice as rich in protein as wheat. Both grasses can be juiced and the juice is extremely beneficial.

Wheat Grass Juice

The simplest and most natural way to obtain wheat grass juice is to chew small amounts of grass, then swallow only the juice. It is best to use a manual juicer designed especially for grass because its slow rotation prevents oxidation of the juice. These are available from the Wholistic Research Company (see Resources Directory). (The use of a blender or centrifugal juice extractor oxidises the juice which greatly reduces its nutritional value.)

● Simply feed the grass into the receptical and the juice will flow out of spout. The machine ejects the dry pulp and it need only be cleaned once per day.

● Let the juice sit for a few minutes after juicing so that the sediment settles in the bottom of the glass. Do not drink the sediment.

● Mixing sprouted seeds, celery, parsley or spinach with wheat grass makes the juice more palatable but use small quantities of the grass during each feeding of the machine. One box of wheat grass, which is properly planted and cared for, can produce up to 2½ lb of grass, and 1lb of seeds will produce about 4lb of grass. With the correct grass juicer it is possible to extract at least 10 fl. oz of juice from one pound of grass. Harvesting should begin between the seventh and fourteenth day of planting.

Growing your own wheat grass

Obtain two large, heavy duty plastic trash bags and fill one with the best available compost. Add more compost to a plastic tray 9.25 x 5 x 2 inches or thereabouts and then sprinkle some crushed kelp with your fingertips onto the soil and mix it in well. Plant the wheat seed shallowly, lightly covering it with soil and put the tray into the trash bag which will create a greenhouse effect. Keep the tray in a window and after three days remove the covering.

Somewhere between the seventh and fourteenth day the grass will be at least seven inches high and ready to harvest. After the first harvest the second growth of wheat grass is still worthwhile, but the third growth is of little value.

After harvesting the grass, store the sod in the second plastic trash bag by placing the first mat root downwards and all the others root upwards. Then drop a few earth worms into this, closing the bag very loosely so that the worms are able to breathe. In three to six weeks the sod will break down into soil which can again be used for planting.

When using wheat or barley grass juice for the first time it is a good idea to take it in very small quantities, perhaps only a tablespoon. Take enough to make you feel uncomfortable but not so much that you feel like vomiting it up again. Both are powerful cleansers because of their high enzyme contents, so they will start immediate reactions with toxins and mucus in the stomach, often causing nausea. This feeling of nausea merely proves that they are needed and should be taken regularly. Thirty minutes before drinking any of the juice, drink a quarter of a lemon squeezed into a glass of water, or, if you have an acid stomach, a glass of mint tea. Both methods will clean out mucus from the stomach and minimise discomfort.

Grass juices in 1 or 2 fl oz (30/60 ml) doses can be taken immediately before sprouted seeds. Try to take any grass juice on an empty or nearly empty stomach. That way it is immediately absorbed. Diluted or undiluted rectal implants of wheat grass juice can be used and are often much easier to absorb than taking it orally. The correct amount for a rectal implant is 4 fl oz. Use 1 or 2 fl oz of pure wheat grass juice diluted with 2 oz of purified water. Raw grass juices can be used as a mouthwash. Remember chlorophyll will bring oxygen to the mouth and this is particularly helpful for anyone who has thrush or candida in their mouth or throat.

PURPLE DULSE, KELP AND OTHER SEAWEED

Norwegian Seas are amongst the cleanest in the world, try and buy seaweed from Norway. Of all the seaweeds dulse has the richest mineral concentration but I particularly like it because it tastes bland. I find many other types of seaweed, including kelp, taste rather fishy and as I am a vegan I find it offensive. All sea plants contain the minerals and trace minerals that are found in the oceans and the earth's crust and are easily assimilable.

All seaweeds are a rich source of organic iodine valuable in overcoming poor digestion and goitre, and in re-building and maintaining the function of all the glands. They are useful as an adaptogen in thyroid disease of any description.

BEETROOT

Beets change inorganic raw elements into plant materials that are easily assimilated by us. Beetroot is particularly famous for its blood-building ability. It can be used as part of an anti-cancer diet and is a superb liver and blood cleanser. Raw grated beets and their juices were once used to treat TB, obesity and gonorrhoea. The anthocyans, or plant pigments, in beets are particularly helpful in alleviating symptoms of radiation poisoning.

DARK GREEN LEAFY VEGETABLES

All dark green leafy vegetables, especially spinach, are high in calcium, iron, vitamin K, and of course chlorophyll. If you are juicing any dark green vegetables use the juice in very small quantities as it is extremely potent (see the section on grasses for information on how to juice). The organic oxalic acid found in raw leafy vegetables such as beet greens, Swiss chard, kale, turnip greens, broad leafed sorrel and spinach is excellent for treating constipation. However, once cooked the oxalic acid can settle in the joints, so if you are prone to gout or rheumatism don't eat these vegetables cooked.

In the 1950s the British Ministry of Health and Public Service Laboratory accepted that spinach juice, cabbage juice, kale and parsley juices were far superior to milk for relieving excessive production of hydrochloric acid in the stomach.

ROSEHIPS, ORANGE AND LEMON PEELS

These are some of the best sources of vitamin C and contain the whole vitamin C-complex including bioflavonoids, rutin, hesperidin, calcium and all the trace elements that are now known to be necessary to assimilate vitamin C. All citrus peels contain pectin which is known to remove heavy metals such as mercury and lead from the body, and even radioactive contamination like Strontium 90. When you eat citrus fruit always eat some of the white pith as it contains the bioflavonoids.

BIOFLAVONOIDS

The bioflavonoids in the pith of citrus fruit is highly active and unstable and easily destroyed by heat and exposure to the air. Some of the bioflavonoids, particularly quercetin, are extremely active against viruses including herpes. Nobiletin is powerfully anti-inflammatory and the rutin present in buckwheat lifts depression as well as acting as a preventative against bruising.

Certain bioflavonoids are believed to be anti-carcinogenic and one complex – methoxylated bioflavonoid – stops red blood cells clumping together, decreasing blood viscosity by as much as six per cent.

Bioflavonoids are at their most powerful and active when the body is under stress which is why many of them are useful for combating fungi, viruses and bacteria.

NON-ACTIVE SACCHAROMYCES CEREVASIAE NUTRITIONAL YEAST

There are literally hundreds of different types of yeast available but many on the market today are the by-products of manufacturing processes in the brewing industry (hence the name brewers' yeast) or designed for the baking industry. These yeasts are often used as food supplements. My feeling is that their nutritional value is suspect and their quality is poor; some may even be toxic. Nature gives you a clue because potentially harmful yeasts often taste and smell somewhat unpleasant and bitter. Importantly some are still active, meaning alive, and can be damaging to those people who have yeast infections such as Candida albicans.

Saccharomyces cerevasiae nutritional yeast is grown solely for human consumption as a nutritional food supplement. It is cultivated on a base of pure beet and cane molasses and it absorbs this base in the same way as plants utilise minerals in the soil. Molasses is used because it provides the yeast with an abundant organic source of B vitamins and minerals. Once the yeast is harvested it is thoroughly washed and dried and during the drying process it is heated just enough to stabilise it, so making it completely non-fermentable. This process not only makes the yeast incapable of any further fermentation in the digestive tract but helps it to be easily digestible and absorbable. It is therefore particularly recommended for those with internal bacterial or fungal infections, including Candida albicans.

GARLIC

Garlic, known botanically as *Allium sativum*, is certainly one of nature's miracle foods. The ancient Egyptians, Greeks and Romans all used garlic copiously to increase their strength and fight disease and illness. Hippocrates used garlic specifically to treat cancer. In the First World War the British government used garlic in battlefield hospitals to disinfect and heal internal battle wounds. It was also administered to treat typhoid fever and dysentery.

Today garlic is the leading over-the-counter drug in many European and Asian countries. It is an official drug in many countries, such as Japan, and is prescribed by medical doctors outside the US for many diseases, especially hypertension (high blood pressure) and high cholesterol, as a broad spectrum antibiotic, antiviral agent and fungicide. It can be used as part of an anti-cancer diet.

Garlic is famous for its healing power with respect to heart disease. Countries where garlic consumption is high are shown to have a lower incidence of heart disease than average.

Garlic lowers serum cholesterol and triglyceride levels and reduces the build-up of atherosclerotic plaque in our arteries. It does this partly by increasing the blood levels of HDLs. These lipoproteins clear the blood of excess cholesterol and fat. Garlic also lowers LDLs which can attribute to arterial plaque. Medical researchers have also found substances in garlic that inhibit blood platelet aggregation (the sticking together of blood cells). Garlic also reduces hypertension.

One third of all the medical research into garlic is cancer related. The National Cancer Institute in America has reported that cancer incidence worldwide is lowest in the countries where garlic consumption is highest. Garlic has been shown to help white blood cells combat cancer and increase the ability to destroy tumours. When chemicals derived from garlic are present in the bloodstream, many aspects of our immunity are enhanced. Garlic has also been found to stimulate interferon production, enhance natural killer cells, stop tumour growth, and even reduce the associated pain of cancer. Garlic has been found in double-blind studies to reduce the incidence of colon-rectal cancer and stomach cancer. With over eighty different sulphur compounds, it is a free radical scavenger. This is just another way that garlic protects from cancers, even those that are chemically induced.

Garlic is a powerful antibiotic, antiviral and antifungal agent. Garlic juice diluted one part in 125,000 has been found to inhibit the growth of bacteria. In Russia it is so revered as an antibacterial agent it has been christened 'Russian penicillin'.

Garlic is selective in its bacteria destruction, only killing bacteria that are harmful. At the same time garlic actually enhances helpful bacteria and improves our intestinal flora and digestion.

Garlic acts against many types of bacteria including streptococcus, staphylococcus, typhoid, diphtheria, cholera, bacterial dysentery (travellers' diarrhoea), tuberculosis, tetanus, rheumatic bacteria and many others.

Garlic is a powerful antiviral agent and many feel it could be the cure for the common cold. It attacks the different viruses that cause upper respiratory infections and influenza. Garlic has been shown to destroy on contact the viral agents responsible for very many diseases.

Garlic's antifungal ability is second to none. Laboratory tests have proved it to be more potent than any known antifungal agent. Garlic will regulate the overgrowth of Candida albicans.

● THE IMPORTANCE OF FOOD COMBINING ●

It was in 1902 that Ivan Pavlov, in his ground-breaking book *The Work of the Digestive Glands'*, conclusively proved that every kind of food stimulates a specific definite type of gastric and intestinal secretion. So if you want to absorb your food properly and make full use of it, it needs to be ingested in specific and optimum combinations. If you don't do this the partially digested food can produce harmful toxins which place strain on a body trying to off load the poison. Besides which, the one process that uses the most energy in our body is digestion. It takes up more energy than running, swimming or cycling. So if we treat our digestive processes kindly our organs will not be prematurely exhausted.

Different kinds of food need different types of digestive juices and not all of these juices are compatible. Starchy foods (rice, barley, wheat and potatoes) need an alkaline environment for digestion whereas proteins (nuts, soya beans) need an acid solution. If you mix a starchy food and a protein together (dates and nuts, eggs and french fries, beans on toast) both acid and alkaline digestive solutions are simultaneously produced. They neutralise each other and digestion grinds to a halt or is impaired. The starches ferment causing a souring of the stomach and gas. If you keep this up you may develop a stomach ulcer.

If you wake up exhausted after seven or eight hours of solid sleep every night you may well be hypoglycaemic (see p. 33) but you may simply feel that way because your digestive system has been overloaded with trying to digest the incompatible mess inside you. This can go on for fourteen hours. Properly combined foods digest in only three or four hours.

SOLUTION

- Try to eat only one concentrated food in a meal, that is any food that is not water-rich. Water-rich foods embrace **all** fruit and vegetables except squashes, pumpkin, potatoes and legumes which count as concentrated foods because they are more dense and solid. Concentrated foods include meat, fish, eggs, cheese and rice.
- Do not eat protein and starch mixed together.
- Do not mix fruit and starch. In fact **all** fruit should be eaten in isolation and on an empty stomach. This is because it is high in water and as such is cleansing, leaving behind no toxic residue. It is easy to digest. In fact it doesn't digest in the stomach it is partially predigested by the enzymes in the saliva in the mouth and sweeps through the stomach in twenty minutes releasing its supercharged nutrients into the small intestine and the bloodstream. Fruit juice acts even more rapidly as an energy boost. This applies to fresh fruit and freshly squeezed juices. Baked, canned, stewed or dried fruit does not have the same nutrient value, nor does cooked or chemicalised juice. Allow twenty to thirty minutes to pass before eating or drinking anything else and wait three to four hours if you have previously eaten anything other than fresh fruit.

• CYCLICAL EATING •

Our bodily rhythms are circadian. The eliminative organs, particularly the liver, are working flat out at the complex processes of detoxification from 4 a.m. until midday. Why then would you want to interrupt this vital process with an improperly combined hearty traditional breakfast? The sensible thing to do is to have only fresh fruit, fresh juices and herbal teas till midday. If you suffer from morning sickness or hypoglycaemia you may like to add nature's Superfoods to your juice (see p. 25–31) and then to sip ginger tea with honey and lemon to still the nausea.

From midday until approximately 8 p.m. is the most suitable time for taking food. If you eat a very late meal you will feel uncomfortable.

Your body assimilates food best between 8 p.m. and 4 a.m. providing the food is properly combined. If it isn't digestion will take a lot longer than that. If you are hungry in the night, eat any amount of fresh fruit and juices but **nothing else**.

Initially all of this may seem mind-bogglingly complicated but please try it and see. Just observe the simple food combining rules and I **guarantee** your energy will rocket.

• WATER WITH MEALS •

Do not drink water with your meals as it dilutes and weakens the digestive process. Carbonated water may taste more exciting than plain water, but carbon dioxide is a waste gas which your lungs are constantly breathing out so why cram it into your digestive tract? It will cause wind, discomfort and burping.

Since water makes up eighty per cent of your body, your diet should consist of lots of water-rich foods and pure water. Water-rich foods are fresh fruits and vegetables and their freshly squeezed juices, as well as fresh sprouts. Other sources of water include soya milk, nut milks, rice milk, herbal teas, coffee substitutes and, of course, pure water itself. Water-rich foods are designed to cleanse and nurture your body simultaneously. The cleaner your body the more effectively it will work for you.

• QUALITY OF WATER •

Millions of people in Britain drink water contaminated with toxic chemicals at levels which are sometimes in excess of international standards. Over 350 different man-made chemicals have been detected in British tap water.

FLUORIDE

About ten per cent of the people in the UK and fifty per cent in the USA drink fluoridated water. Some research has indicated that high levels of fluoride might be associated with cancer, genetic disorders, brittle bones and mottled teeth. The problem is most of us over-consume fluoride from natural sources, such as food and drink, as well as being exposed to artificial sources like insecticides, anaesthetics and preservatives. The difficulty is that only half of all ingested fluoride can be excreted by the average healthy adult. Children, diabetics and those with debilitated kidneys may retain as much as two-thirds of their ingested fluoride. In extreme cases this build-up in the body may be associated with bone-related cancer, liver/bile cancer, oral lesions, abnormal cell changes and metaplasias (replacement of one tissue type with another). The link between fluoride and brittle bones has long been established but even very low levels of fluoride inhibit the ability of leucocytes (infection-fighting white blood cells) to migrate, which means fluoride depresses the immune system.

Unfortunately there are, as yet, no filters on the market able to remove fluoride so if you live in a fluoridated area I suggest you drink bottled spring water. There is a machine which removes all chemicals from water but it is expensive and makes the resultant water taste very flat .

• COFFEE •

The incidence of pancreatic cancer is low, but coffee drinkers are at least twice as likely to develop it than those who abstain, and the rate is directly proportional to the amount consumed. Coffee is rich in oil and most pesticides are soluble in oil, so the high rate of pancreatic cancer found in coffee drinkers might be a result of high exposure to pesticides. The caffeine in coffee is linked to heart disease and coffee drinkers who drink up to five cups a day suffer from more heart attacks than non-coffee drinkers. Coffee can cause palpitations, high blood pressure and raised cholesterol levels. It can also increase acid secretions in the stomach, aggravate fibrocystic breast disease and in extreme cases slightly increases the risk of miscarriage and birth defects. It can aggravate insomnia, anxiety, panic attacks and depression.

Decaffeinated coffee is not the answer. Trichlorethylene was used to decaffeinate coffee until quite recently when it was discovered to be carcinogenic. Now petroleum-based solvents are often used and my feeling is that these too will almost certainly be proved to be harmful. The only firm I know which does not use chemicals and which is prepared to divulge exactly how their decaffeinated coffee is produced is Nestlé. They have told me that their beans are flushed several times with pressurised hot water which dissolves the caffeine. This then drains away in the liquid. The green beans are then washed and marketed as freeze-dried instant coffee called 'Descaf'. If you are a coffee addict you can take this occasionally but even decaffeinated coffee can upset the digestive process because it contains high levels of tannic acid.

The combination of caffeine and sugar in fizzy drinks is particularly insidious because both caffeine and sugar are highly addictive.

The good news is that there are some excellent alternatives on the market including grain coffee made from cereals and fruits, chicory and dandelion coffee. Some dandelion coffee tastes sickly sweet because it is mixed with lactose (milk sugar) and I would not recommend this. It is possible to buy roasted ground dandelion root from medical herbalists and other herbal suppliers. This needs to be boiled up for twenty minutes, using about half an ounce of root to a pint of water and then thoroughly strained before drinking. The added bonus is that it is wonderfully cleansing and strengthening for the liver as well as purifying the blood. Do not mix it with milk – milk makes it taste decidedly odd in my opinion. Try to drink it black and unsweetened because the bitterness is what activates the liver, but if you can't manage it add a touch of honey or maple syrup.

• TEA •

Most people are very surprised to learn that there is twice as much caffeine in tea as in coffee, which makes it a very strong stimulant. The tannin in tea is so astringent that it actually inhibits the absorption of iron, resulting in indigestion and lack of energy. Imported tea sometimes contains copper and other impurities and it is often fumigated with chemicals. Alternatives include Bancha made from the twig of the tea bush which contains no caffeine. Rooibosch tea is made from *Aspalanthus Linearis* and has a pleasant smoky flavour which is rich in vitamin C and trace minerals, whilst being caffeine free. Herbal teas can take a bit of getting used to. However, there are some excellent ones on the market. My favourite brand is called Celestial Seasonings. I make a detoxification tea which actually not only tastes brilliant but works on a medical level (see page 63). Please note that many commercially available herbal teas have no kind of medicinal effect on the body but by drinking them you are avoiding the caffeine and tannin in tea.

• ALCOHOL •

It might be good news to hear that wine and beer are actually believed to be healthy when taken in moderation; no more than two drinks a day, always with meals. Wine is closer in composition to our gastric juices than any other drink, but do be wary. It may also be loaded with chemicals none of which need necessarily be listed on the label.

Many asthmatics react severely to the sulphur dioxide used in wine to halt fermentation and kill bacteria. Other common additives include white sugar as manufacturers are permitted to use up to fifty-three per cent water and/or sugar in wine. It is also legal to use a variety of nearly a hundred additional additives. You can avoid all this by buying organic wines which are becoming increasingly popular (see Resources Directory).

Many beers also contain additives. German beers manufactured specifically to the 'Bavarian purity decree' are excellent and include Lowenbrau, Lederer-brau, Spaten, Wuzberger and Hofbrau Bavaria.

• DIGESTIVE ENZYMES •

I once attended a wonderful lecture given by pioneering nutritionist Jay Kordich who at that time was in his late-seventies but had the energy of a teenager. He had spent forty years promoting the power of freshly squeezed juices all over the USA and his central theme, which he chanted like a mantra was, 'don't eat cooked foods late at night', by which he meant after about seven or eight p.m. He understood the importance of cyclical eating and suggested that if you absolutely had to eat late at night you should sprinkle digestive enzymes made from pineapple or papaya over the food first or scatter the dish with lots of raw chopped onions which are rich in digestive enzymes. When we are healthy our bodies produce their own enzymes for specific jobs like breaking down fats or proteins, but ageing, erratic eating, crash dieting, stress and nutritional deficiencies all take their toll on natural production. The end result can be energy depletion, indigestion, digestive disturbances and food intolerances. For an excellent supplier of these enzymes see the Resources Directory.

• SPROUTED SEEDS •

Sprouted seeds are abundantly rich in digestive enzymes, as well as vitamins, minerals and amino acids. They are power houses of energy. The vitamin E content of wheat grains triples once sprouted, the B2 content of oats rockets by 1,300 per cent. Once a seed sprouts it is in effect predigested and even those with food intolerances can digest sprouted seeds comfortably. Unlike cooked pulses they do not cause wind.

Sprouted seeds are cheap and easy to grow on a windowsill in a large, wide-necked glass jar. Placing them on a sunny windowsill will encourage the production of cholophyll. Simply soak the seeds you want to sprout overnight in purified water. Tip them into a sieve and rinse and drain them thoroughly. Then pour them into your jar and cover the neck with muslin, cheesecloth or a clean pair of old tights secured with a rubber band. Tip the jar on its side and make sure there are no more than two inches of sprouts so they can breath and grow. Rinse and drain the sprouts twice daily and in a few days they will be ready to eat. You can eat them once the root is as long as the seed and for several days afterwards until green leaves begin to appear. Store them in the fridge in a sealed plastic bag or airtight container having rinsed them one last time and drained them thoroughly.

• STRESS AND DIGESTION •

Another of Kordich's themes was that it is not natural to eat cooked food late because it stresses the body at a time when it wants to rest and sleep.

Never eat when you are stressed. We require more than good nutrition to make us happy and healthy. Anger and resentment actually act like physical poisons in the body. Fear can compromise your immune system so much it will finally make you ill.

• SUMMARY •

The heartening but extraordinary fact is that once you cut out all junk food from your diet and clear the rubbish from your system your body will be intuitive enough to tell you what it needs. I know this to be true because I have seen it working with my patients over many years. Somehow the powerful and ancient knowing with which we are born, but which, often during the time in which we grow up, gets buried under a deluge of rubbishy chemicalised food, manages to surface again.

It is certainly true that no one diet is perfect for everyone but my feeling is that a vegan diet is probably the healthiest possible diet for almost everyone. However, I have known some people vomit up even a teaspoon of chamomile tea at the beginning of diet reform. This is not instinctive body talk. It is simply because the body is so toxic and the digestion so distorted and battered that it cannot deal even with the simplest bit of nutrition. If this is the case I will often get the patient to start with just a few drops of certain medicines or teas and graduate from there. Accurate body talk only begins once you have cleaned the body up. While in process the messages can often get very confused. It's a bit like learning to ride a bike. You wobble about a lot and fall off several times but whenever you courageously remount and keep wheeling you eventually get the hang of it and you find the speed, once you know how to manage the bike, is wonderfully exhilarating. At that point you won't have to rely on any books, videos or gurus, you will find exactly what you also wanted to know about what suits **you**.

You know by now that I am not a great believer in shop-bought vitamins and mineral supplements and you will have read about the reasons why. In an ideal world, a balanced diet of fresh unprocessed whole food would supply all our vitamin and mineral needs but unprocessed, unchemicalised food is very hard to come by, and you should always remember that nutritional needs vary greatly depending on age, stress, illness, pregnancy, alcohol and tobacco intake.

One thing I noticed many years ago when I began to transfer my alliegance to an imaginative, balanced, wholefood and largely raw diet, was that my taste buds got sharper and fussier and I actually felt nauseated not just naughty when I ate foods which did not suit me, or I would get headaches, aches and pains, a mild rash, diarrhoea, halitosis or a myriad of other symptoms. I decided it was simply not worth paddling in my own poisons, although from time to time when I fall off the straight and narrow with a resounding crash, I pay the penalty as cheerfully as I can.

CHAPTER 3:

HERBAL PHARMACY

———

• METHODS OF APPLYING HERBS •

This chapter is designed for simplicity. Herbs can be administered in all sorts of ways to help heal illness. They can be smelled, swallowed, injected into any bodily orifice (enema or douche), gargled or applied to the skin. I would remind you that fasting and using water treatments are sometimes the best medicine of all and for these aspects of self-healing see the following chapter, Basic Maintenance.

• WATER-BASED HERBAL PREPARATIONS •

A water-based herbal preparation is any herb prepared in any way with water. (Herbs can also be prepared with other solutions including apple cider vinegar, alcohol and glycerin.)

Internally these are administered as teas; externally as baths, poultices or fomentations. Water will only extract the water-soluble principles of the herbs. If using fresh herbs they should be gently crushed between the fingers, with a stainless steel knife or in a pestle and mortar. Crushing breaks down the cellulose of the plant. Dried herbs may need to be further chopped or pounded in a pestle and mortar. Water-based preparations decompose rapidly so they need to be made freshly every few days. Store any excess in the refrigerator or in a glass jar or china basin covered with muslin or linen to allow the preparation to breathe. If fine bubbles pop up to the surface you will know that your mixture is beginning to ferment so throw it away, preferably over plants in the garden, if you have one.

INFUSIONS

Delicate parts of the herbs including the flowers, leaves and stamens should be steeped in water for twenty minutes using 1 oz (30 g) of the herb to one pint (600 ml) of freshly boiled filtered water. Stir the preparation with anything except aluminium and cover the container tightly leaving it to steep, just as you would a tea, for fifteen minutes, then strain through muslin, nylon or a stainless steel or silver tea strainer.

DECOCTION

The tough parts of the herbs like seeds, roots, barks, berries or very tough leaves like bay leaves all need much more rigorous processing to ensure the active constituents are released into the water, because their cell walls are so strong. Remember all seeds, roots, barks and berries need to be thoroughly crushed in a pestle and mortar or a coffee grinder before use. The only exceptions are burdock root and cinnamon sticks which merely need steeping in freshly boiled, but not boiling, water, and valerian root which should be steeped in cold water for twenty-four hours before being boiled. Decoctions will generally stay fresher longer than infusions.

To make a decoction

Put 1 oz (30 g) of herbs into a glass, enamel or stainless steel saucepan and cover with 1 pint (600 ml) of filtered water and a tight-fitting lid. Bring the mixture to the boil and simmer gently until the water is reduced by half (normally fifteen to twenty minutes). Strain as above and use as required.

• ALCOHOL-BASED HERBAL PREPARATIONS •

Alcohol is a better solvent than water and has the advantage of acting as a preservative. An alcohol-based preparation is called a tincture and these are readily available from health food shops and your local medical herbalist. Tinctures are normally taken internally and diluted in water first but they may be rubbed onto the skin directly or applied on poultices previously dampened with water. When making a composite tincture buy one of each herb and mix them together proportionately. Store in opaque glass, tightly stoppered.

HOW TO MAKE A TINCTURE

Using good quality brandy, gin or vodka (never use alcohol in the form of surgical spirit or methanol as these are poisonous) combine 4 oz (125 g) of powdered or very finely chopped herbs with one pint (600 ml) alcohol. Keep the container somewhere warm; an airing cupboard is ideal. Shake vigorously daily or twice daily if you have the time and strain after fourteen days. You will generally find the final amount of alcohol is only one-third of the original amount as the herbs, which are strained out, absorb much of it.

Tinctures should be started with a new moon and strained with a full moon fourteen days later. The power of the waxing moon helps extract the medicinal properties. Evidence to support this theory is available in *Moon and Plant* by Agnes Fyfe. In this book the author discusses the moon's nodal cycle in relation to both the earth and plants on it. Over many years she conducted 70,000 consecutive single tests on plant sap which proved that the moon had chartable influence on the way sap rises and falls in plants. Her experiments show us that such practices as old herbalists collecting herbs at a particular time are not arcane but vital if herbs are to be used at their most effective. (There are diaries that chart the course of the moon which may be obtained from local metaphysical bookshops.) Once the tincture has been made strain it through coffee filter paper into a labelled bottle and cap it tightly.

• HERBAL POULTICES •

Poultices are a useful form of treatment for external wounds or grazes and for drawing out any type of poison or unwanted material from the skin, such as thorns and splinters. In addition they nourish the skin and can be absorbed into the lymph and blood beneath the skin. Poultices are an excellent way of softening and dispersing material that has become hardened, such as scar tissue. The best time to apply a poultice is before you go to bed at night.

MAKING A POULTICE

You will need
- Fresh herbs which have been liquidised in a little water *or* dried herbs which have been soaked in a little hot water *or* powdered herbs. The herbs you choose will depend on the purpose of the poultice.
- Slippery elm powder (make sure that this is 100 per cent pure slippery elm as the slippery elm sold in health food shops contains only a minute percentage of real slippery elm), cornflower, marshmallow root, or arrowroot as a carrier base.
- Apple cider vinegar.
- White cotton. A large handkerchief is suitable but gauze can also be used.
- Two large china plates and a large saucepan of boiling water.
- Plastic sheeting such as a piece of trash bag.
- A supply of stretchy cotton bandages and safety pins.

Gauge the amount of material you will need depending on the size of area to be covered. A poultice to cover your abdomen will require more than one to cover a spot on your wrist. Estimate how much of the herb will be needed to treat the area in question to a depth of one-quarter inch (6 mm). Put the chosen herb(s) into a basin and add an equal quantity of the carrier base and just enough apple cider vinegar to form a thick paste. Stir the mixture with a stainless steel or wooden spoon. Once thoroughly mixed, place the plate over the saucepan of boiling water and put the square of cotton on top of the plate.

Scrape all of the herbal mixture onto one half of the cotton, keeping it away from the edge to stop it squelching out when you use it. Fold the other half of the cotton over the top and press the edges together. Now cover the poultice with the other plate and boil the water until the poultice has become thoroughly hot. Put on some rubber gloves and remove it.

Apply the poultice as hot as is bearable to the affected area – make sure that it is not so hot that you burn yourself. Now cover the poultice with your plastic, secure with bandages and safety pins or, if the area is very large, a thin towel. Leave it on overnight.

Next morning peel the poultice off and warm it up again using the same plate method. Meanwhile cleanse the area with a mixture of half apple cider vinegar and half purified water. Re-apply the poultice to the area being treated but this time use the other side against the skin. Leave it on all day. Repeat the process in the evening but start with a completely fresh poultice and continue this sequence until the area is healed.

In an emergency simple poultices made by chewing the relevant freshly picked herb into a pulp can be applied directly to the skin.

• HERBAL COMPRESSES •

These are simply thin liquid poultices which are used if large areas are to be treated. They assist the circulation of lymph or blood to a specific area so relieving swellings like varicose veins, goitre, and muscular pain. Cold compresses will ease congestion in the head, insomnia, fever, indigestion, sprains, bruises and sore throats. Hot compresses will relieve any internal congestion over a specific organ.

If you are treating a whole arm or leg with a compress apply it by using cotton tights or a long cotton glove soaked in the herbal mixture. Silk stockings, although difficult to find, can also be used – any natural material will do. Such compresses are very effective for treating varicose veins, thread veins, eczema, psoriasis and ulcerous conditions.

I am very keen on compresses in my own practice although I sympathise with patients going to bed accompanied by the unglamorous rustle of a trash bag!

MAKING AND APPLYING A HOT OR COLD COMPRESS

A compress can be made from fresh, dried or powdered herbs, oils, plant juices or tinctures diluted in water.

Make a double strength herbal decoction or infusion by using 2 oz (60 g) of your chosen herb to one pint (600 ml) of water. Strain the mixture then dip a cotton cloth into it and wring it out lightly but firmly. If the mixture is hot protect your hands with rubber gloves. Wrap the part to be treated with the compress and secure with bandages, covering these with plastic wrap or a piece of plastic which will keep the moist heat of the compress intact and protect clothes and bed linen from seeping dampness. If you are sleeping in the compress you may also need to protect your mattress with a piece of plastic. The compress should only be kept on for as long as it remains hot. It can be kept hot longer by placing a hot-water bottle over it. Alternatively, it can be renewed if you have a second hot compress ready to use.

If the compress needs to be re-used, the simplest way is to turn on a slow cooker or a saucepan, fill it with your herbal decoction or infusion and drop in the damp compress. Leave the lid off. The compress will heat up again very quickly and if frequent changes of compress are needed they can each be kept hot and within reach.

Cold compresses are made in exactly the same way but the liquid is allowed to go quite cold before the cloth is dipped in. A cold compress will encourage the blood to move quickly to the surface in cases of high temperature, sprains and bruises. It should be applied for five to fifteen minutes and if it is being used to reduce a fever it will be necessary to change the compress every five to ten minutes as it heats up. A cold compress left on for half an hour will relieve indigestion (if placed over the stomach) and insomnia (if placed over the forehead or around the back of the neck) and may be repeated if desired once every two hours. A cold compress left on the throat all night will relieve a sore throat and bring down a swelling or swollen joints if placed over the affected area.

• CASTOR OIL FOMENTATION •

A fomentation is simply the technical term for a poultice to be used over a large area. A castor oil fomentation is something I frequently recommend.

The medical properties of the oil of castor beans have been recognised for thousands of years. I have found castor oil applied directly to liver spots a superb way of clearing them up. Coupled with dietary control castor oil has eliminated fatty lumps and calcium spurs under the skin, and applied to the nipples of breast-feeding mothers it has increased lactation. One of my patients healed her husband's diabetes using a castor oil fomentation faithfully and consistently for six months, and another got rid of the warts on her back.

Prepare a fomentation as you would a poultice, by heating the castor oil up first in a (not iron or aluminium) saucepan. The castor oil fomentation can be used three or four times before a new piece of cloth needs to be employed.

• VAGINAL DOUCHES •

These reduce the instance of non-specific vaginitis and relieve painful periods. In good health the vagina is self-cleansing so douches should only be used on a temporary basis and even then no more than two douches a day should be taken. The addition of a tablespoonful of apple cider vinegar or a teaspoonful of freshly strained lemon juice to every two pints (1.2 litres) of herbal infusion or decoction will help to maintain the natural pH balance of the vagina.

Your douche kit should be kept scrupulously clean and it should not be shared with anyone else.

HOW TO TAKE A DOUCHE

1. First make an infusion or decoction, depending on the parts of the herb to be used, then strain it through muslin or coffee filter paper. (An infusion is always made with only flower and leaves whereas a decoction is made from hardier parts of the herb including the roots, bark and berries.) Allow your herbal mixture to cool to body temperature then fill the douche bag with it.
2. Hang the douche bag (the ones I sell have a strong hook attachment) on the wall over your bath at shoulder level. Now climb into the empty bath and lie down. If the bath is cold, warm it up first by running hot tap water around it and letting it drain out.
3. Lying on your back insert the nozzle slowly and gently into the vagina until it touches the cervix and then slowly release the closed tap on the douche bag allowing the herbal tea to flow into the vagina.
4. With both hands seal the vaginal opening around the nozzle so that the vagina becomes flooded and balloons open with the herbal mixture. If you are doing this correctly you will feel a slight sensation of pressure as the vagina opens to accommodate the fluid.
5. When it feels full, shut the tap with one hand while you release the hold of the other hand so allowing the vagina to drain. The liquid will come out fairly rapidly.
6. Repeat the whole procedure until all the herbal tea is used up. Douching while standing up is a complete waste of time.

Pregnant women should never douche and should not douche for at least four weeks after delivery. Women who experience pain while douching should stop at once. Persistent vaginal infection should be reported to a doctor.

• ENEMAS •

My female patients often fear enemas. If they have experienced an enema at all it is usually just before childbirth, administered amidst fear and discomfort and often using soapy water which induces violent and painful peristalsis (as well as destroying all the benign bacteria from the colon). Let me reassure you. An enema is really easy and comfortable to administer if you do it correctly. All you have to do is allow yourself plenty of time and privacy and lay out everything in advance because the more relaxed you are the easier you will find the whole process.

Let me dispel another myth. Enemas do not make a mess. Your anal sphincter is quite capable of holding liquid in the colon until you decide to release it. Initially it is common for the stimulation of the enema fluid on the bowel to make you want to rush straight to the toilet and release it but you will acquire self-control with practice.

Taking an enema is really quite logical. You wouldn't dream of unblocking a drain from the top end of the waste pipe. Using the same analogy a blocked colon needs to be relieved from the bottom end. In the event of a fever an enema is the quickest way to relieve the bowel of toxic waste. If you are so weak you cannot eat then an enema can supply nourishing superfoods to the digestive tract. Colonic irrigation which uses fifteen gallons of water to wash out the colon, administered gently and a little at a time, is thirty-two times more powerful than an enema. For a list of colonic therapists see Resources Directory.

> *Enemas should never be relied upon to replace your usual bowel movements, nor should they be abused by over use. It would not be acceptable to take an enema everyday to remedy constipation, for example. I would consider this over-use. Enemas are excellent to take waste out of the system in an emergency, such as a high fever, headache, etc.*

If you are pregnant or suffer any serious bowel disease consult a doctor before administering an enema.

You will need:

- Three and a half pints (2 litres) of a herbal decoction or infusion made with filtered water. Cool enemas are used for cleansing, and warm ones for treating nervousness and spasms.
- An enema kit (see Resources Directory).
- Olive oil, Vaseline or KY jelly.
- A large bath towel or a piece of plastic sheeting.

HOW TO TAKE AN ENEMA

1. Fill up the enema bag with your chosen infusion or decoction at the right temperature and hang it from a hook in the bathroom at shoulder height.
2. Lubricate the tip well with Vaseline, olive oil or KY jelly.
3. Place your towel or plastic sheet on the floor and lie down on your right side with your knees tucked up to your chest and gently push the lubricated tip of the enema tube into the rectum. It won't slip in too far because it is joined to the kit with a tap which acts as a barrier.
4. Release the tap and allow the liquid to flow slowly into the rectum. If the liquid encounters a block of impacted faeces you will feel marked internal pressure, so turn off the tap and massage the area in an anticlockwise direction.
5. When you have used half the enema liquid, carefully roll over onto your back with your knees bent and place the soles of your feet flat on the towel or plastic sheet beneath you. Release the tap. When the enema pack is emptied of its contents turn off the tap and remove the nozzle tip.
6. Carefully stand up and wrap yourself in a bath towel then go and lie down on your bed with your bottom raised on some pillows. If you are nervous about spilling any of the enema mixture onto your bed cover the bed first with a plastic sheet.

7. Retain the enema for twenty minutes if you can. Get up and release whilst sitting on the toilet.

• HERBAL OILS •

These are easily obtainable from health food shops and your local medical herbalist. Garlic oil can be bought in capsules, as can borage and evening primrose oil.

• OINTMENTS AND CREAMS •

Again these are easily obtainable from your health food shop and local medical herbalist. Ointments are particularly effective for dry and cracked skin and need to be applied generously and rubbed in thoroughly. Creams are better for treating sore, chapped skin and protecting and moisturising healthy skin because they are lighter and more easily absorbed. Their moisturising effect is enhanced if you spray the skin first with a flower water or diluted apple cider vinegar.

• PESSARIES •

For suppliers of T-Tree pessaries see Resources Directory. Applied vaginally they are useful for treating thrush and applied anally they are useful for treating haemorrhoids and systemic candida. Pessaries should be used every night, one inserted before going to bed and renewed nightly for a week, to do their work well (see Resources Directory).

• SYRUPS •

These are readily available from health food shops and your local medical herbalist will stock certain syrups, but they are easily made at home.

To a strained decoction add one-quarter of its weight in liquid honey, then stir it over a low heat until the honey is dissolved. You may need to skim off the rising scum from time to time. Alternatively you can mix one-quarter part of tincture with the equivalent weight of honey and combine the two over a low heat. Decant into a labelled glass bottle. Syrups are an excellent basis for cough mixtures, and are very pleasant gargles if diluted in their equivalent weight of hot water.

• DRY PREPARATIONS (POWDERS) •

These are probably the most potent and effective form of herbal medicine because the whole herb is used, not an extract. However, their disadvantage is that when powdered leaves and flowers are exposed to oxygen and moisture which quickly break down important active constituents, they have a maximum shelf life of a year. Powdering does not break down the cell walls which are difficult for our digestive systems to process, so they are not recommended for those with poor digestion. Powdered herbs are usually packed in capsules, very few of which are now made out of animal products, but in some instances it is essential to taste the herb, as when taking bitter herbs. Their effectiveness depends on the sensation of bitterness stimulating the digestive process. If you need to taste the herbs, powders are best put into a little warm water and drunk. You can buy herbs already finely powdered from the suppliers listed in the Resources Directory.

• CAPSULES •

These are available in sizes ranging from 00 to 4. 0 is the correct size for an adult. To fill the capsule simply separate it and press each half firmly into the powdered herb until it is as full as possible. Then close the capsules so that one side slots into the other. The normal adult dose would be two or three size 0 capsules with a meal. If you have difficulty in swallowing capsules but can manage tablets, or vice versa, you need to look at your swallowing technique. Place a tablet or pill in your mouth with a small amount of water and tilt your head right back. You will find that you will swallow the tablet readily. Follow with more water. This method does not work with capsules, because they are lighter than water and so will float forward and be difficult to swallow. Instead tilt the head and the whole of the upper body forward so the capsule floats back as you swallow easily. For suppliers of capsules see Resources Directory.

• PILLS •

These are readily available in health food shops. Avoid those with brightly coloured sugar coating.

• DOSAGES •

As a general rule the dose of any herb should follow body weight. The doses I give throughout this book are for adults weighing 150 lb (75 kgs). In my clinical experience I have found that people who are underweight, highly strung or both should spread the dose on a continual basis throughout the day and that alcoholics and drug addicts need higher doses than would be expected from their body weight, at least until they have completely detoxed. Alcoholics should never be given herbal tinctures.

> *Herbs should not be taken while fasting unless otherwise instructed by your professional medical herbalist.*

● STORING HERBS ●

Anything made into a tincture will keep up to eight years if stored in firmly stoppered opaque bottles in a dark cupboard. Dried herbs will store well for one year only. Honey is an excellent preservative so syrups will store well for several years. Herbal oils will keep indefinitely if stored in small, sterilised, opaque glass bottles and if used infrequently air gaps should be eliminated by transferring them into smaller and smaller bottles as they get used up. Poultices and compresses should always be freshly made and the cotton and gauze bandages should be boiled well after use, dried and stored in sealed brown paper or plastic bags. If they have become sticky with ointment thrown them out.

● SUPPLIERS ●

Bioforce: I have dealt with this company now for many years and greatly admire the fact that by and large they are unique among herbal manufacturers for using only freshly harvested herbs in their tinctures. The herbs are cultivated in a remote north-eastern corner of Switzerland between 800 to 1,500 feet about sea level which encourages the condensation of the healing properties in them. In other words they have to be hardy and powerful to survive at this height. This company is also particularly rigid about harvesting according to strict protocols. For example, echinacea purpurea is harvested when it reaches three to four feet in height when fifty per cent of the flowers are in bloom and fifty per cent are in bud. Harvesting takes place after midday for two reasons. Firstly, the dew will have evaporated from the herb, so stopping the possibility of mildew, and secondly, the sap rises highest in herbs at midday.

While many professional herbalists in practice, including myself, are particularly keen to harvest their own herbs freshly whenever possible, most commercially available herbal tinctures are not manufactured to Bioforce's particularly high standards. All Bioforce's products are readily available in health food shops.

Nature's Plus: This company does extensive third party testing on all their products. It is highly recommended by many health food store owners.

Earthrise: Sell very high quality spirulina, chlorella, barley and wheat grass.

Butterbur & Sage I have not encountered essential oils commercially available which are made to the extremely high standards this company employs, and most experienced aromatherapists tend to agree with me.

Nelsons: Make a superb range of herbal ointments and creams. I particularly like this company because they use as much fresh base herb as they can. Scientific testing using chromatography proves that fresh herb preparations contain more of the active constituents and are more stable compared to their counterparts manufactured from dried herbs.

• THE SAFETY OF HERBS •

Not all herbs are benign and beneficial. Many plants have not yet had their bio-chemical qualities, whether toxic or therapeutic, fully documented. What constitutes a toxic dose of a normally therapeutic herb depends largely on circumstances. The toxic dose may be 300 times the medicinal dose and herbs in this quantity would be extremely difficult to ingest. However, there are herbs that have a toxic dose so close to the therapeutic one that any attempt by the amateur at self medication could end in disaster. I have listed all these herbs on pages 50 to 51. Warnings to pregnant women are in bold-type.

Remember it is always best to treat an acute condition without any herbs at all. *Fasting is the best medicine of all.* **If in doubt about any aspect of herbal medication please consult a professional, qualified medical herbalist.**

• POTENTIALLY DANGEROUS •

This is a checklist of herbs that are not suitable for use in home treatment. Read through it carefully before taking any of the herbal medicines in this book.

ACONITE

There are some thirty species of aconite, all containing the deadly poisonous alkaloids *aconitiny* and *pseudoaconitine*. If these are ingested in anything but the most minute quantities the results are fatal. **Please do not use this herb at all**.

ALOE

Aloe vera and aloe gel are both potent in their action and should **never** be used internally. A cut leaf of aloe from the living plant rubbed externally over burns, rashes, psoriasis, insect bites and itching is extremely helpful but if you ingest the **whole plant** it will cause internal ulceration and piles. However, the juice taken internally and under the supervision of a medical herbalist can be used to heal internal ulceration.

Normally the dried sap of either Curacao, Barbados or Cape aloes are used internally but they need to be mixed with herbs to counteract the griping effect on the bowel. **Aloe should never be used by pregnant women**.

BAYBERRY BARK

See *Sage*.

BELLADONNA

This should **only** be used by **qualified medical herbalists** as it is part of the Solanecae family and one of the better known plant poisons.

BLACKBERRY

See *Sage*.

BROOM

This should **not be used if there is high blood pressure or during pregnancy**.

BUTTERCUP

The sap is extremely dangerous taken orally.

CAYENNE PEPPER

Always take cayenne pepper uncooked. It can cause burning on defecation but this will be helped by mixing it half and half with slippery elm.

CELERY

Celery seeds are often treated with a poisonous fungicide so buy organic celery if you possibly can. **It is a uterine stimulant and so should be avoided during pregnancy**.

CHAMOMILE

People often think of this as the gentlest of herbs but I have observed that strong infusions can cause nausea, so take in small amounts at first.

CLEAVERS

See *Sage*

CLOVER

Some varieties of white or Dutch clover contain hydrocyanic acid which can break down into prussic acid in the digestive system and become extremely poisonous. Ensure that you use red clover only. If using clover on the skin it is advisable to mix it into a carrier base such as slippery elm or marshmallow, as prolonged contact can cause burning and soreness.

COLTSFOOT

Coltsfoot contains pyrrolizidine alkaloids **and should be strictly avoided during pregnancy**.

CRAMP BARK
This relaxes the uterus so should not be used during pregnancy.

COOKED SPICES
Most spices if cooked, as in a curry, aggravate the digestive system. They are much more therapeutic if taken uncooked (see Cayenne Pepper).

FALSE UNICORN
This contains substances which mimic a hormone that helps bring on labour **so it should not be used during the course of pregnancy** (see pages 20–23). However, taken under supervision it is a superb herb for inducing fertility in women, as it is one of the most stimulative tonics to the uterus and ovaries. It can be a gastro-intestinal irritant in large doses.

FOXGLOVE
If taken in excess it is deadly so it should not be used by amateurs.

GARLIC
Garlic eaten raw is very beneficial for high blood pressure but processed garlic in the form of pearls or tablets can actually aggravate the condition. Chew a raw clove after eating garlic to fresh your breath.

GINSENG
This is best used in chronic diseases where the patient is weak, cold and debilitated. **It should never be given to those with acute hot fevers, those suffering from high blood pressure, or to women with menstrual irregularities**. Nor should it be taken with anything containing caffeine. For the older person or for prolonged treatment of debilitation, the maximum dose is 800 mg of the dried root daily. The young and active should not take it for more than three weeks and should then discontinue treatment for at least two weeks. The maximum dose for the young and active is 2 grams daily. This advice applies to Asiatic ginseng (Panax ginseng) and American ginseng

(Panax quinquefolium). Siberian ginseng (Eleutherococcus senticosus), although a member of the ginseng family, has a different kind of action. Extensively researched in Russia, and given to 20 million Russian workers on a regular basis, it has been proved to be the best of all the adaptogens. It can increase the productivity and learning capacity of the brain and combat fatigue. It can also modulate stress hormones, so helping the body to adapt to non-specific stress. It is excellent for blood sugar regulation, jet lag and chronic tiredness. Siberian ginseng is a worthwhile herb to take in tincture form whenever you feel under stress.

GOLDENSEAL
This should not be used by diabetics because it lowers blood sugar levels. If it is taken for more than three consecutive months a previously unaffected person may begin to exhibit the symptoms of diabetes. Taken long term it will stop the absorption and digestion of B vitamins in the digestive tract. **It should not used during pregnancy because it contracts the uterus**. However, in non-pregnant women it is an excellent antibiotic if used short term.

GREATER CELANDINE
In large doses Greater Celandine is extremely poisonous. Its sale is restricted to medical herbalists only.

GROUNDSEL
Excessive use over short periods of time may cause cirrhosis of the liver.

HAWTHORN BERRIES
These are not to be used if you have a low blood pressure.

HEARTSEASE
Excessive doses can cause a cardiac reaction. **Take this only under the supervision of a medical herbalist**.

HEMLOCK

Hemlock is poisonous. Avoid Cicuta, waterhemlock, which is equally fatal.

HOLLY

The leaves are sometimes used to treat rheumatism but the berries are poisonous. Make sure no one nibbles them over Christmas.

HORSETAIL

This should always be used with a demulcent herb to soften its effect. A demulcent herb is anything that is very high in mucilage. This is the softer, fleshier part of the herb. Slippery elm and marshmallow are excellent examples. Horsetail contains silicic acid, saponins, alkaloids and a poisonous substance called thiaminase which causes symptoms of toxicity in both humans and animals. Thiaminase poisoning causes a deficiency in vitamin B and can lead to permanent liver damage.

JUNIPER BERRIES

Juniper berries are wonderful for clearing up a brief attack of cystitis but should only be used for this kind of emergency, never for prolonged treatment.

LIME TREE FLOWERS

Always ensure your supplies are fresh. Old fermenting leaves and flowers can cause hallucinations.

NUTMEG

This should not be used during pregnancy because it can cause abortion. It is perfectly acceptable to use in small quantities in cooking but in large quantities the poisonous alkaloid, strychnine, can result in fatalities.

PENNYROYAL

The essential oil can cause abortion and should be avoided by pregnant women. The powdered herbs or leaves made into a tea are much milder and can be used in the last six weeks of pregnancy (see page 131).

PEPPERMINT

See Sage.

PILEWORT

This should never be ingested fresh or rubbed on to the skin fresh because it causes irritation. Once dried the toxins in the plant break down making it safe to use.

POKE ROOT

The leaves are extremely poisonous. They contain mitogenic substances, that is substances that distort cell structure. Poke root should be taken under the guidance of a medical herbalist. Properly administered it is an unbeatable cleanser for the lymph and the blood, and is excellent for chronic catarrh and benign cysts.

RED RASPBERRY LEAF

This contains fragine which strengthens the uterus but cannot promote uterine contraction unless a woman has a genetic background of strong pelvic muscle. In other words if a woman has a damaged pelvic muscle, or a genetic weak constitution, red raspberry leaf will not make things better. However, for the average woman it is excellent. Its high iron content makes it one of the favourite herbs during pregnancy but it is best administered with the same quantity of another herb (see Pregnancy Tea Formula p. 126).

RUE

If inhaled in large amounts it is hallucinogenic.

SAGE

Because it is rich in tannin Sage should not be used for a prolonged period of time. Tannin builds up proteins and eventually reduces the absorption of B vitamins, interfering with the absorption of iron. Very prolonged use of any astringent herb that contains tannin has been associated with throat and stomach cells becoming cancerous, so herbs rich in tannin are all best used only for the short term. These include Bayberry Bark,

Blackberry, Sarsparilla, and Yellow Dock as well as Peppermint, Cleavers, and Uva ursi.

Sage also contains a toxic ketone as part of its essential oil complex, and if the essential oil is consumed regularly over several months this may produce womb spasms and the possibility of abortion. Sage oil is therefore not to be used by pregnant women.

SARSPARILLA
See *Sage*.

SASSAFRAS
The oil is carcinogenic so use the whole herb. **Do not use during pregnancy. Do not take for longer than three consecutive weeks even if you are not pregnant.**

SHEPHERDS' PURSE
This is not to be taken during pregnancy because it stimulates the uterus.

SQUILL
This can cause drastic diarrhoea and re-tching and must be given only by a qualified medical herbalist.

ST JOHN'S WORT
Taken internally in tea or tincture form St John's Wort can cause skin reddening and soreness in susceptible individuals.

The oil used externally on the skin can cause puffiness and swelling. Avoid sunbathing while using this herb in any of its forms.

TANSY
This should not be used during pregnancy as it stimulates the uterus.

TOBACCO
Avoid at all costs.

VALERIAN
Valerian should not be taken for long periods because over time it can cause degeneration of the nervous system.

VIOLETS
Always use the fresh and not the dried flowers, as the dried violet flowers are bereft of most of their healing properties which reside in the fresh essential oil.

WHITE BRYONY
In large doses it is toxic.

YARROW
This causes uterine contractions and should not be used in pregnancy.

YELLOW DOCK
See *Sage*.

• WARNING ABOUT ESSENTIAL OILS •

It takes 7,000 or more flowers to make a single drop of undiluted essential oil so you should treat all essential oils with a great deal of respect. Taken incorrectly, some oils can be dangerous in some circumstances to this applies to both their internal and external use. If in any doubt at all consult a qualified medical herbalist or aromatherapist.

• POISONING BY PLANTS •

IF YOU SUSPECT RECENT POISONING

Seek immediate medical help. Keep the patient calm. Panic only increases the speed at which a poison will invade the system. Don't clear up any vomit until the doctor has inspected it. Undigested plant material in the vomit can give important clues about the nature of the toxic material swallowed.

CHAPTER 4:
BASIC MAINTENANCE

───

• FASTING: THE ULTIMATE DETOX •

Fasting is undoubtedly the most powerful medicinal tool I use in my practice. Most therapeutic fasts last from three to seven days. The only liquid taken is mineral or purified water and fruit or vegetable juices and broths decocted from them.

Fasting helps the body to heal itself by allowing the digestive tract to rest, by encouraging the mobilisation of various detoxifying defence mechanisms and by stimulating consequent recuperation. The theory behind fasting is that the body is well equipped with mechanisms for eliminating nutritional waste and also the toxic effects of negative feelings which can be argued to cause more illness than any other factor. Our digestive process uses up thirty per cent of our entire body's energy so if the digestive system is allowed to rest completely that energy can be channeled to detoxification and healing. Fasting is a superb tool both in emergencies and to accelerate the healing of long-term illnesses. If carried out on a regular basis it can help to rebalance the body mentally, spiritually, physically and emotionally. Fasting is also an invaluable preventive medicine. Not only does it help the body achieve peak physical fitness by periodically unburdening itself of accumulated waste, it also prevents minor health problems developing into major ones. Fasting also decelerates the ageing process, and helps the body to utilise nutrition far more effectively after the fast is broken. Research has shown that if juice fasting is done on a regular basis it can achieve remarkable results including faster healing and a greatly reduced risk of DNA damage, the enhanced ability to fight off cancer-causing substances and even helping to promote longevity. The uninitiated often think fasting will lead to stress and fatigue but in fact it does quite the opposite. I have found it the most potent quick-acting antidote to lethargy and anxiety. I always emerge from a three day or longer fast looking younger, with better skin, with my hair and nails in better condition, a few pounds lighter and with abundant energy.

WHEN NOT TO FAST

The following people should not fast.

- The very elderly, fragile or emaciated.
- People with weak hearts.
- People suffering chronic anxiety, depression or phobias.
- Pregnant women.
- Anyone suffering a longer term chronic illness requiring continued medical supervision, whether orthodox or complementary.

HOW DOES FASTING WORK?

One-quarter of your body cells are growing, half are at the height of their working powers and the remaining quarter are dying and being replaced. Only by the speedy and efficient elimination of these dead cells can the building of fresh cells be stimulated. Fasting accelerates the elimination of dead cells and speeds up the production of new, healthy cells. You would think this impossible, because so little nourishment is taken (in a water fast none at all) but it is a proven physiological fact. Meanwhile, protein levels in the blood remain constant and normal because proteins are constantly decomposed and resynthesised for alternative use. The building blocks of protein – amino acids – are released and reused in the process of building new cells, while the cleansing capacity of every eliminative organ in the body is enhanced. Toxic waste in urine has been measured as increasing up to ten times during a fast and an overburdened liver can dump its waste six times more quickly than usual, especially when the fast is enhanced by hydrotherapy.

HOW TO FAST

I mentioned juice fasting because I suggest that you never fast on water alone, especially if this is your first fast. The first fast is a miserable experience for bodies groaning with toxins from our polluted environment and contaminated foods. Toxins pour into the system so rapidly that you may feel like you are drowning in your own poison.

A juicer is one of the first tools I insist anybody working with me purchases. I call the juicer 'nature's intravenous drip' because fasting with juicers can alter the quality of the bloodstream more rapidly than any other method available. Juices bought from health food stores and supermarkets tend to be boiled and so leached of many of their nutrients, or they have preservatives added to them. Anything which is bottled and labelled organic is generally acceptable, although there are juices that are organic but contain whey. While fasting on these is better than not fasting at all, I would urge you to find a source of organic fruit and vegetables and juice them freshly as needed.

WHEY

Whey is a by-product of cheese production. I think it looks like pus, tastes appalling and stinks. Only ten per cent of the milk used to make cheese actually ends up as cheese. The rest separates out as whey and the cheese industry has to dispose of it somehow. Whey is so toxic it cannot be poured into sewers and very few ordinary sewage works are capable of treating it. Dumping it into streams merely leaches out all the oxygen and kills the fish. Put into land fills it may seep into water supplies. Nevertheless, whey is found not only in some bottled juices but in baked goods, ice-cream, luncheon meats, substitute chocolate, soup mixes and chocolate beverages.

Home-made juice

Freshly pressed home-made juice is particularly beneficial because you can drink large quantities and therefore absorb more vitamins, trace elements, minerals and enzymes. Fruit juice helps to maintain a stable blood electrolyte balance so ensuring that the circulation remains constant, but water alone has the dangerous capacity to distort circulation. Besides all this, juices are easily digested. Within fifteen minutes of being swallowed they are absorbed into the bloodstream. They do not stimulate the secretion of hydrochloric acid in the stomach, a particularly important point for those with ulcers or tender stomach linings. They contain an unidentified factor which stimulates the micro-electric tension in the body which is responsible for the cell's capacity to absorb nutrients from the bloodstream and so promote the effective excretion of metabolic waste. This is very exciting news for cellulite sufferers. Cellulite is partly the result firstly of the colon failing to dispose of waste as efficiently as it should and secondly of poor lymphatic drainage so that wastes become trapped in spaces between the cells. Juices' ability to cleanse the lymph and bloodstream rapidly helps to disperse cellulite. For those with heart and circulatory problems the concentrated sugars in juice actually strengthen the heart.

How much juice should you take?

When supervising patients through juice fasting it is often difficult to get them to drink enough juice. You should aim to drink one fluid ounce (30 ml) of juice for every pound (roughly 500 grams) of your body weight every day. This means that you may well be drinking up to a gallon (4.5 litres) of liquid a day. The more liquid you ingest the quicker you flush out all those accumulated toxins and the less possibility there is of retaining water, because mineral water or purified water and juices act as natural diuretics.

How to juice

All juices should be served at room temperature and, if possible, pressed freshly as needed (to minimise oxidation) and they should be well 'chewed' before swallowing. You don't actually have to move your jaw to do this. Just swish them around your mouth to ensure they are mixed with plenty of saliva before swallowing.

When juicing, remove the skins of such fruit as oranges and grapefruits because they contain toxic substances that should not be consumed in large quantities. However, leave on the white pithy part of the peel because it contains valuable bioflavonoids. Tropical fruits such as kiwi and papaya should be peeled before pressing because they are grown in countries where carcinogenic sprays are still legal and still used. The skins of all other fruits and vegetables including lemons and limes can be left on, but if the fruit has been waxed remove the peel. All stones should be removed before juicing but seeds can be placed in the juicer with the fruit. Those fruits and vegetables that contain little water, for example, bananas and avocados, cannot be juiced but can be used as an ingredient in a fruit smoothy. A fruit smoothy is fresh fruit juice liquidised with fresh and frozen fruit. My favourite recipe is 8 fl oz of apple juice liquidised with one fresh banana and a cupful of frozen berries at high speed until the whole mixture is creamy.

Before juicing wash all your produce well and remove any mouldy or bruised parts. Throw the excess pulp onto your compost heap if you have one. If you have to prepare juice in advance, store it in a thermos flask and fill it as near to the top as possible so there is no air left in the flask, adding the juice of a lemon to stop oxidation. Try to make juice only from locally grown produce in its proper season. Juice will keep adequately in a thermos flask without fermenting for up to eight hours.

Potassium broth is a very useful addition to a fast (see page 15). Do not mix fruit and vegetable juices together as the enzymes in them are incompatible. The only exception to this rule is carrot and apple juice. Various types of juice will heal specific conditions – further information is given in the bibliography.

STARTING AND FINISHING A FAST

- Ease into and out of a fast by eating fresh fruits and vegetables for one, two or three days beforehand and afterwards. Never shock the body by changing from a heavy diet to fasting or vice versa unless you are fasting for emergency first-aid purposes.
- If you have never fasted before fast for between one and three days only. Fasting for longer than a week needs supervision from a professional experienced with the technique.
- Breaking a fast is as important as the fast itself. You can undo most of the good gained by a fast by breaking it improperly or unwisely. It is best to break a fast by eating a home-made vegetable soup containing some well-cooked grains or by eating fresh fruit and, separately from the fresh fruit, a large raw salad lightly dressed with olive oil and lemon juice. Spend as long breaking a fast as the fast itself. So if the fast took three days, introduce solid foods gradually over a three-day period.
- Do not be too rigid about how long you fast. I have started three-day fasts and gone on for ten days because I was feeling so wonderful; I have also

set out to do seven-day fasts and finished after thirty-six hours because I had had enough. Fasting has the advantage that it requires less time spent on menu preparation than normal eating patterns required (providing you haven't bought dirty carrots and have to spend all day at the sink scrubbing them) and eliminates the possibility of choice and hence temptation.

- Fasting for more than a day actually lowers the metabolic rate and the spectacular amount of weight that is lost during the initial days of a fast is merely the result of the liver disposing of glycogen and water levels adjusting in the body. A substantial percentage of the weight lost during a long fast is rapidly regained after normal eating has been resumed, which is reassuring news for very thin people, but not good for fat ones.
- However, fasting, for those who want to lose weight, is a wonderful introduction to controlled eating because it shores up willpower and shrinks the stomach so that smaller helpings suffice, and because digestion of any food eaten after a fast is greatly enhanced and hormonal secretions are stimulated.

SUPPLEMENTATION AND DRUGS DURING FASTING

If you are taking drugs prescribed by a doctor, do not start a fast without taking his or her advice. If you are taking any natural medicines under the supervision of a complementary practitioner, do not start a fast without telling him or her. In either case, your fast might need supervision by a naturopathic professional.

Any vitamin and mineral supplementation during the fast is inadvisable for reasons stated on page 24. The exceptions to these are the Superfoods listed on pages 25–31. These are as easily ingested as juices themselves, so place no extra burden on the digestive system. I have found spirulina, chlorella and nutritional yeast particularly helpful for stopping blood sugar swings during the first three days of a fast, and for appeasing the appetite. Use them in copious quantities if desired. You can take up to six or seven heaped teaspoons a day of spirulina and chlorella, liquidised into your juices. Stirring merely leaves unappetising green lumps floating on the surface. You can take four dessert spoons a day of nutritional yeast. This is particularly good stirred into potassium broth (see p.15 for recipe).

WHAT TO EXPECT DURING THE FIRST THREE DAYS OF A FAST

It is common to experience symptoms such as dizziness, mild heart palpitations, weakness, lightheadedness, tiredness, forgetfulness, mild nausea, a nasty taste in the mouth, a furred tongue, and a gnawing or empty feeling in the stomach and abdomen. If these do happen just take extra rest, detach yourself from anything negative that floats through your mind, inspire yourself and shore up your willpower by reading books on fasting (see Bibliography). **But never try to pep yourself up with stimulants during the course of a fast.**

All the unpleasant physical symptoms that may be experienced during the first three days of a fast are the result of toxins being eliminated. The more fasts you do the less likely it is that you will experience these. During a prolonged fast it is very common to experience a 'healing crisis'. This usually begins on the tenth or eleventh day and may manifest itself in a variety of ways, ranging from flu-like symptoms to skin eruptions and other eliminative processes. A healing crisis is to be welcomed with joy (although you might not feel like doing so as you are going through it!).

If you are worried by unpleasant symptoms, or they are persistent or unusual, stop the fast and seek professional advice.

FASTING AIDS

Skin brush regularly (see p. 61), morning and evening, and wear only natural fabrics at all times. Remember to sleep in cotton sheets. Walk barefoot on grass, sand or soil for five or ten minutes every day. Air bathe for a few minutes daily, exposing the whole body naked to the air while lying in the shade. If it is icy or snowing outside, air bathe by standing naked in front of your open window. Fresh air accelerates wound healing and encourages the skin to breathe properly. Take time to breathe properly and deeply (see p.64).

Stay with the natural rhythm of the day, getting up when the sun rises and taking a rest shortly after it sets. You will probably find you need extra sleep during a fast, at least in the initial stages. Try and fit in some extra rest before midday when the liver is still very active. The liver bears the brunt of cleansing during a fast and is at its most active between 4 a.m. and midday. Some time between these hours apply a castor oil poultice to the liver and lie down. By lying down you will increase the blood flow to the liver by forty per cent and the castor oil pack boosts this flow by a further twenty per cent.

Take an enema before bed every day of your fast. This is by far the quickest and most efficient way to cleanse the colon (see p. 44). Alternatively, if you are on a long fast and know a good colonic therapist, have a colonic irrigation two or three times a week. I am one of the few colonic therapists in Britain who offer Dr. Bernard Jenson's deep tissue cleansing management programme which involves a colonic every day, together with an enema morning and evening. You would be surprised at the amount of waste that is disposed of on this programme. A lot of people fasting on juices get complacent and think the colon will have nothing to excrete, but one of its functions is to act in much the same way as the skin, drawing waste from the blood and lymph system through the intestinal wall.

Don't watch television and be selective about the things you read. Your favourite poetry, inspirational books about health, healing and fasting and books that make you laugh are all fine. Fasting is also a form of spiritual cleansing and if you fill yourself with mental rubbish it will leach your emotional energy and may even give you nightmares. I have found that one of the great things about fasting is that my senses become heightened as my body cleanses itself. My taste buds pick up every tiny nuance of flavour and my sense of smell becomes very sharp. Colours get brighter, sounds more distinct and my sense of touch becomes much more sensitive.

Exercise daily, preferably by taking long, brisk walks well wrapped, unburdened and breathing deeply. As your metabolic rate drops your lymphatic system will slow down but skin brushing and walking will speed it up again and help it to gather up waste and dump it more efficiently.

• SKIN BRUSHING •

The benefits of skin brushing must be tried and tested to be believed. You will feel clean, refreshed, much more alert and ready to cope with anything!

Our skin is the largest organ in our bodies. It flushes toxins outward by way of perspiration and absorbs nutrients and vitamins from natural sunshine. The skin also breathes and absorbs oxygen while exhaling carbon dioxide formed in tissues. The thousands of sweat glands which should operate to expel at least one pound of waste products daily, regulate body temperature and act as miniature detoxifying organs working to cleanse the blood and free the system of suffocating poisons. For all these reasons, it is worth taking special care of your skin.

Skin brushing stimulates the circulation, helping to pump the blood down through veins and up through the arteries feeding those organs of the body which lie near the surface. It also stimulates the lymph and the adrenal glands. It has a powerful rejuvenating effect on the nervous system because of the hundreds of nerve endings in the skin.

The major lymph nodes are dumping stations for waste fluids and you can stimulate the expulsion of mucoid lymphatic material or impacted lymph (cellulite) by skin brushing. These lymph nodes are situated behind the elbows and knees, under the arms, either side of the throat and especially in the groin. Skin brushing removes dead skin layers and other impurities, thus keeping the pores open and unclogged, and increases the eliminative capacity of the skin. Used in conjunction with hot and cold showers skin brushing will help to stop colds from developing.

Five minutes of energetic skin brushing is equivalent to thirty minutes of jogging as far as physical tone is concerned. It will build up healthy muscle tone and stimulate better distribution of fat deposits. All in all it can help you to feel younger and gives a terrific sense of wellbeing.

SKIN BRUSHES

You will need a natural bristle brush with a detachable long wooden handle. You should not share a skin brush, nor lend yours to other people.

At my clinic I sell brushes made with Mexican tampico fibres which I import from Germany. The bristles are quite stiff to begin with, but soften with use. See the

Resources Directory for advice on buying a skin brush. Nylon and synthetic fibres **won't do** as they will create static in the body.

As skin brushing involves using a dry brush on dry skin it is important to maintain the brush properly. Wash it out once a week in warm soapy water, using natural soap. Rinse it well and dry thoroughly.

HOW TO SKIN BRUSH

- Make sure your skin is dry. Start with soles of your feet. Brush upwards towards the heart from below and downwards the toes from above.
- Brush vigorously up the legs and over thighs remembering to brush towards the groin where the lymph nodes lie. Use a circular clockwise movement over the abdomen, following the line of the colon. Do this about ten times. Avoid the genital area and the nipples.
- Brush your palms and the backs of your hands, up the arms to your shoulders. Use downward strokes on your neck and throat and over your chest. To stimulate the lymph nodes under the arms you need to use your hands to create a pumping action. Lodge the thumb under your shoulder bone and with all the fingers grip your chest muscle making sure the fingertips get right into the armpit. Squeeze and then release this area about fifteen times on each side.
- Attach the handle to the brush so that you can brush across the top of your shoulders and upper back, then up over the buttocks and lower back. This should take you about five minutes daily. First thing in the morning is the best time. Should you need to brush twice a day, don't brush too close to bedtime or you will not sleep. Brush every day for three months then reduce it to two or three times weekly, changing the days each week.
- The scalp can be brushed to stimulate hair growth and to get rid of dandruff or impurities but you may prefer to massage the scalp with your fingertips to move the scalp skin.

Do not brush on the face; a softer and smaller brush is needed for that area.

Never brush skin that is irritated, damaged or infected, or over bad varicose veins.

SHOWERING

After your five minutes of skin brushing you should remove the dead skin cells by showering.

- Take a hot shower or bath for two to three minutes followed by a cold shower for twenty seconds, and repeat.

- Move the shower head from your feet upwards and finish by holding it over the back of your skull, letting cold water run down your spine.
- This method of hydrotherapy will alkalise the blood, clean the head and give a special boost to the lymphatic system and vital functions of the body.

You can do several things to look after your skin.

1. Use only natural fabrics next to the skin, for example cotton, linen, silk or wool. Wear only gloves and shoes made of natural fibres or leather.
2. Use only natural organic soaps or olive oil-based soaps and natural oils. These penetrate the skin whilst mineral or synthetic oils only lie on the surface.
3. Take regular exercise to promote breathing. Turkish baths and saunas also help.
4. Encourage eliminations by dry skin brushing daily. When fasting skin brush twice daily, morning and evening.

• A THREE-DAY FAST •

Having been on a light diet of raw foods only the day before, on your first morning of the fast and every morning thereafter do half an hour of deep breathing and stretching, then take a liver flush.

THE LIVER FLUSH

Liver flushes are an excellent way of stimulating the elimination of wastes from the body by opening and cooling the liver and increasing the bile flow, so improving overall liver function. They also help to purify the blood and the lymph. Various preparations are effective as liver flushes, but this is my favourite.

Take one or two cloves of crushed garlic and one inch of finely grated ginger. Liquidise them at high speed into 8 fl oz of juice and add between one and four tablespoonfuls of organic olive oil. The juice you choose can be a combination of freshly squeezed citrus juices, including lemon and lime, or apple or carrot, or carrot and beetroot juice. Both ginger and garlic have been proved to have excellent liver protective qualities in recent studies in Japan. Garlic provides important sulphur compounds that the liver needs to build enzymes (see Paracetamol in the Appendix on Drugs).

Follow the liver flush with two cups of hot detox tea or two cups of peppermint tea, using 1 oz of peppermint leaves soaked for 20 minutes in one pint of freshly boiled water in a covered vessel. Alternatively, peppermint tea bags bought from a health food store would also be suitable.

Detox Tea

Equal parts of:
roasted chicory
roasted dandelion root
licorice root
ginger

coriander seeds
orange peel
hawthorn berries
cinnamon sticks
carob pods

Decoct and drink hot. This tea detoxifies the liver and cleanses the blood; it supports the kidneys, facilitates digestion and strengthens the heart.

Do not eat or drink anything for one hour after your liver flush. If possible, use the time to lie down with a castor oil poultice over your liver. When the hour is over drink 8 fl oz of prune juice. If you make it yourself, soak ten organic prunes in two glasses of water overnight. Liquidise in the morning but, remember to take the pits out. Prune juice has an extraordinary ability to draw toxins from every part of the body and eliminate them through the bowel, which is why bowel movements after prune juice often smell so strange and so strong.

Half an hour after taking the prune juice, drink 8 fl oz of another juice, diluted half and half with still mineral water or purified water. Continue taking the mixture at half hourly intervals through the day.

Choose one juice for each three-day period alternating between fruit and vegetable juices so that you maintain a balance between cleaning and regeneration.

You may take potassium broth instead, particularly if your body temperature is dropping and you are beginning to feel cold (see p.15 for recipe). Herbal teas may also be taken freely throughout the day. You may continue with your detox tea or use any other herbal tea.

Take an enema before bed and don't forget to use all your other aids during fasting.

I would remind you once again to break your fast wisely.

KIDNEY CLEANSE

In order to cleanse the kidneys choose water melon juice, if it is in season. Include some of the seeds and one square inch of rind in every 8 fl oz of juices. If water melon is not in season, use grape juice instead. Potassium broth should be alternated with every glass of one of these juices. If you want to cleanse your kidneys, on rising take seventy drops of the following kidney/bladder tinctive in one pint of warmed water containing the juice of a freshly squeezed lemon, followed by two cups of kidney tea.

Kidney/Bladder Tincture

2 oz/60 gm dandelion leaf
2 oz/60 gm uva ursi leaves
1 oz/30 gm of each of the following:
juniper berries
corn silk

horsetail
gravel root
burdock root
`golden rod flowers

See page 40 for instructions on how to make a tincture.

Kidney/Bladder Tea

Equal parts of:
dandelion root
horsetail
uva ursi leaves

chamomile
buctin
nettles
meadowsweet flowers

*Infuse and drink hot. You should urinate much more copiously on this fast, which
is all to the good.*

LYMPHATIC CLEANSING

The lymphatic system is the body's vacuuming system. Lymph is closely married to
mucus and blood, but unlike blood it does not have a heart to act as a pump, relying
instead on the action of muscles and lungs to stimulate flow through a one-way
valve system. The lymph nodes are concentrated in the groin, behind the knees, in
the armpits and under the chin but they spread throughout the body via a network
of tiny tubes covering every area except the central nervous system. They are full of
white blood cells designed to attack and ingest invaders and to clean out waste.
Differing cells have differing roles. The B-lymphocytes produce antibodies which
immobilise any invader, whether it is from chemical or bacterial sources. The T-
Cells pursue foreign invading cells, fungi, bacteria, viruses and allergens. Between
them they act as a good policing team ensuring that your immune system is doing
what it should. If they falter the lymphatic system clogs up and one or more of the
lymph nodes swells with poisonous waste. You may feel a lump, or see an enlarged
mole. At this stage your lymphatic system needs vigorous attention. It has particular
difficulty in combating heavy metals and industrial chemicals whether they are
eaten, absorbed from the air or rubbed on the skin.

Deep breathing

Deep breathing is one of the most effective methods for cleansing the lymphatic system. This is the breathing that Yogis call *prana yama*. It simply means breathing in as deeply as possible, raising the abdomen while doing so, so that the air reaches the bottom of the lungs, then holding the breath for a specified period of time and breathing out in a controlled way. The best ratio is to breathe in to a count of eight, hold to sixteen and breathe out to a count of eight. Do nine of these breaths a day. Liver and kidney flushes cleanse the lymphatic system too, as does fasting. Manual lymphatic drainage (MLD) is a superb way of encouraging the proper flow of the lymph system but there are very few trained therapists around. (For a list of properly trained therapists see Resources Directory.)

GALL-BLADDER FLUSH

This is recommended only for those who are already experienced with fasting and cleansing. It is an extremely strong cleanse and should not be attempted without the supervision of a medical herbalist.

This flush activates the liver and gall-bladder even more strongly than the liver flush and toxic waste released during fasting will be effectively eliminated. People often eliminate green putty-textured stones. I have often observed a lot of anger, negativity and frustration purged during the course of a gall-bladder flush. I have also seen people who do gall-bladder flushes in groups behaving as if they were drunk. Whether this is due to old drug residues being re-experienced as they are eliminated from the body or the result of a systemic hormonal reaction, doesn't really matter. Either way the gall-bladder flush is an extremely powerful and effective cleanse for liver and gall-bladder.

At 7 p.m. on the third day of your fast, liquidise one pint of organic olive oil with the juice of nine freshly squeezed lemons and take five tablespoonfuls every fifteen minutes.

Even if you find yourself vomiting oil, continue to take it. Sucking an ice-cube or sipping a little decocted ginger tea in between doses of oil and lemon juice often helps with nausea. If you are in any way worried or frightened by the nausea, abandon the flush.

There are some people who find it truly horrendous to drink olive oil in such large quantities, so I suggest they sip it through a child's straw so that it does not contact the lips and goes right down the back of the tongue and throat easily.

Once you have finished drinking the oil, lie on your right side with your knees tucked up and your hips elevated and stay in this position for at least two hours, unless you are actually sitting up to drink the olive oil and lemon juice. Meanwhile distract yourself with some of your favourite music or a good television video if you can see it from this angle.

Once the oil is finished go to bed with a warm castor oil compress over your liver and a hot water bottle. If you need anything else to drink sip only ginger tea or water.

The next morning take a chicory enema or a warm water enema with the juice of a half a lemon squeezed into it. A chicory enema is made as a decoction, 1 oz of root boiled in one pint of water for 20 minutes. Allow the decoction to cool naturally and then strain it and use at luke-warm temperature. Both enemas will help to stimulate elimination but the chicory is more effective. People bring me gifts of what they consequently produce in jars and the gall stones range in size from gravel to beans and seeds, and lumps the size of golf balls. If stored in a jar they will dissolve within a couple of days. In order to retrieve them for your own interest or for your practitioner you will need to wash the bowel movements with running water through a sieve, so go to the toilet in a potty!

This cleanse should only be done once a year and should always be preceded by at least ten days of the liver flush.

• CLEANSING THROUGH THE COLON •

Colon rectal cancer is one of the commoner types of cancer and kills thousands of people each year. Hundreds of thousands of people suffer from other colon disorders. Everyone has experienced some type of bowel disorder, generally constipation. The fact that thousands of tons of laxatives are sold all over the Western world each year confirms this.

There are many reasons why people are getting more constipated, the first being ignorance of proper bowel functions. No bodily function is more subject to extraneous influence than defecation. We tend to suppress the urge to move our bowels and have done so for so many generations that as a society we no longer know what is normal. In primitive cultures where people live in harmony with nature, eat natural foods in season, get plenty of exercise and generally live less stressful lives, bowel problems are far less common.

One of the inhibitions of civilised culture is the thought that moving our bowels is somehow dirty. Among most civilised cultures the anus, rectum and bowel are only second to the sexual organs as dirty, nasty, sinful parts of the body. Whether it be conscious or subconscious, most of us feel some embarrassment or guilt or difficulty about our bowels. Most of our cities are lacking in public toilet facilities. Where there are public toilets, these are often filthy or are centres for all manner of unsavoury activities. Banks, post offices and building societies refuse to supply public toilets. Many restaurants, petrol stations and shops demand that you buy something before they let you use their facilities. The problem of finding a toilet when you need it is, it seems, universal. I find the best way round this is to use hotels, and to walk quietly in as if I am staying there. So far I have never been stopped.

Modern lifestyles have wreaked havoc in our colons. Refined, processed, low-fibre foods and saturated fats, scanty exercise and rising levels of stress have all contributed to the rise in digestive disorders of all types.

It is, in fact, perfectly normal and healthy to have a bowel movement for every meal you eat, so that if you eat three meals a day you could be having three bowel movements a day. According to a standard textbook for the diagnosis and treatment of disease, nearly eighty per cent of people over the age of fifty have diverticular disease. Diverticula are small secular herniations through the wall of the colon. They can become filled with faecal matter and ulcerate, leading to perforation and leakage. This results in the spillage of faecal matter into our abdominal cavities, creating infections. The textbook suggests that populations with a high instance of colon rectal cancer consume diets containing less fibre, grains, vegetables, fruits, nuts and seeds, and more animal and protein fat and refined carbohydrates, than populations with a low incidence of the disease. A sluggish bowel retains pounds of old toxic and poisonous faecal matter and often it is the stubborn retention and reabsorption of this toxic waste that is the cause of disease.

FOOD

I have already made it clear in Chapter Two that a diet of fruits, vegetables, grains, nuts and seeds promotes proper bowel function, but what kind of foods create constipation? The real culprits are foods that have a binding nature, for example meats, dairy products and highly refined foods – all have little or no life in them. Wheat flour, for example, was used for years as wallpaper paste. White glue is a by-product of the dairy industry and is made from proteins in milk. The walls of Venice, which have been standing for over 800 years, were made originally of dirt and eggs.

EXERCISE

Exercise is also a vital factor in good bowel health. The improved circulation and lung capacity produced by exercise, together with the strengthening of abdominal muscles, all stimulate the peristaltic action of the bowel. Peristalsis is a wave-like movement by which waste matter travels through and eventually out of the colon.

EMOTIONS

Together with the food we eat and our exercise programme, our emotions dramatically affect our bowel's ability to perform. Fear is linked with constipation. Whenever you are fearful you create constipation. A constipated and crystallised thought process creates a constipated person.

CONSTIPATION: A SUMMARY

GENERAL FACTOR	Specific cause	Prevention and cure
Food	Meat and all animal products eggs, dairy products and any highly refined food.	Eat fruits, vegetables, grains, seeds and nuts instead.

Liquid	Not enough liquid, dehydrated foods.	Drink one gallon of liquid every day by way of water, herbal teas and fruit and vegetable juices.
Movement	Sedentary lifestyle with a lot of sitting or lying down.	Try deep breathing and exercise, especially abdominal exercise. Even walking can work wonders.
Emotion	Fear, or negativity, holding on to problems, holding on to old, useless material possessions.	Letting go of people and things, open up your mind, become an open, aware and loving person.
Drugs	Any drugs which sedate or are narcotic. Opiate derivations such as codeine.	Try digestive stimulation and cathartic herbs.
Intestinal Flora	Antibiotic drugs, extremely hot food, loud noises over seventy-two decibels, X-rays, sudden violent changes in the weather, being bottle fed as a baby.	Instead take fermented nuts, seeds, grains and vegetables such as sauerkraut. Positive ions. Breast feed from birth. Garlic.
Toilet	Sitting upright on a Western-type toilet necessitates pushing down against the rectum and positively encourages haemorrhoids.	Squatting with your feet elevated on a box or a pile of magazines ideally raised to within six inches of the toilet seat, with your knees spread and your elbows resting on them is the ideal way to take a bowel movement. This position relieves the bearing down on rectal muscles.

FRIENDLY BACTERIA

Every colon holds three to four pounds of resident bacteria as indigenous flora. This is made up of three or four hundred different species of bacteria whose activities have wide-reaching effects on our metabolism, physiology and biochemistry in ways that are both beneficial and harmful.

These micro-organisms can be either indigenous or transient. The former colonise the intestinal tract by sticking to the gut lining; the latter are ingested in food and drink and are constantly in transit from the mouth to the anus. Together they make up nearly forty per cent of the whole weight of our faecal matter.

The bacteroids, together with coliform bacilli and E-coli, are the putrefactive bacteria responsible for the decaying matter in the colon. They enjoy a diet full of protein and fat which accelerates the output of undesirable metabolites like bile salts, urea, phenols, ammonia and other dietary degradation products which are all potentially harmful substances, doubly so if there is already constipation or a malfunctioning liver present. A high population of bacteroids bacteria is one of the main contributory factors to the development of degenerative diseases such as ulcerative colitis, diverticulosis and haemorrhoids. Unfortunately, most people have a ratio of eighty-five per cent of these potentially harmful bacteria to only fifteen per cent beneficial bacteria.

The beneficial bacteria produce acetic, lactic and formic acid which acidify the intestine, so preventing the colonisation of fungus like Candida albicans. When the percentage is better balanced peristalsis is stimulated, flushing out toxic bacterial metabolites and waste products in the faeces and so checking putrefactive bacteria.

Intestinal flora

Some foods promote benign intestinal flora such as natural, raw, unsalted, sauerkraut, miso soup and fermented grains like Rejuvelac, as well as some herbs, especially garlic. Garlic is capable of destroying harmful bacteria while encouraging good bacteria.

The most vicious destroyers of beneficial intestinal flora are antibiotics. Whether we consume them as by-products of the meat or dairy industry or take them for infections, all antibiotics cause enormous quantitive as well as qualitative changes in the intestinal flora, creating a perfect seed bed for pathogenic micro-organisms and actively encouraging the growth of Candida albicans.

Radiation of the abdomen even with X-rays upsets the normal microbial balance of the colon, as do sudden violent changes in the weather and loud prolonged music above seventy-two decibels.

Stress

Stress has a profound effect on intestinal ecology. It doesn't matter what the source of the stress is; the stress response stimulates the release of adrenalin and cortisol as the body alerts itself for 'fight or flight'. These hormones then induce a number of physiological changes, including the drying up of oral and gastric secretions, the retention of sodium chloride and the acceleration of potassium excretion and raised blood sugar. Cumulatively these reactions alter the intestinal habitat, decreasing the micro-organic goodies and increasing the baddies. When you consider how much routine stress you are exposed to, ranging from bright lights, atmospheric pressure, noise and crowds and how much more is self-generated from fatigue, anger, anxiety, pain and fear, it really makes you appreciate just how hard it is to generate the right sort of balance of intestinal bacteria.

QUANTITATIVE AND QUALITATIVE ANALYSIS

How often do you have a bowel movement and exactly what should it look like? This is a subject most women would prefer not to discuss. Many people have a library in their bathroom; if you have time to read while sitting on the toilet it is a sure sign of constipation.

Having a bowel movement should be easy, comfortable and quick. When you feel the urge, you should be able to evacuate your bowels in less than two minutes and be finished, without straining, squeezing or grunting. Every bowel movement should be soft and mushy like cottage cheese, slightly gaseous and should crumble and break up as it reaches the water in the toilet. If it is well formed or any harder or dryer than this you are constipated and could fall victim to haemorrhoids. Remember, ideally you should be having a bowel movement for every meal you eat, but in no case, even when fasting, should you have less than two a day.

HERBAL HEALTH

There has been much controversy over both cathartic and laxative herbs over the years. Many of my patients are worried about becoming addicted to natural or chemical laxatives, and this is certainly possible, but only if they neglect a natural food programme, emotional healing, and a good exercise programme. When my patients adjust their attitudes, closely follow a natural food programme and take exercise they have been able to wean themselves off laxative or cathartic herbs completely and enjoy natural bowel movements every day. I am somewhat bemused by this fear of becoming addicted to laxative herbs, especially when I consider the alternative. The side effects and outcome of constipation can be disease in any part of the body, but especially in the colon.

The following suggestions will help to promote better bowel elimination. I begin with minor methods working up to stronger steps towards the end.

1. Drink a minimum of one gallon of water, herbal teas or diluted juices every day. Dehydration of faecal matter is a major factor in chronic constipation. It is very hard for dried-up faecal matter to travel through the colon, and liquid simply hydrates it and makes peristalsis easier.

2. Cathartic fruit juices such as prune and fig have long been famous for their bowel-cleansing abilities, but apple juice is also quite effective, as is pear juice. Prune juice has the ability of drawing in waste through the colon wall from the surrounding bloodstream, so this is particularly recommended. Drink up to two quarts daily, preferably freshly juiced and well 'chewed', served at room temperature.

3. Mucilaginous herbs like phyllium seeds and flax seeds are capable of absorbing many times their natural weight in water and so bulk up in the colon and act like a soft sponge to push faecal matter through and encourage peristalsis. Flax seeds are also rich in their own natural lubricating oil.

4. Both cayenne pepper and ginger root greatly increase bowl activity. Work up to taking at least one rounded teaspoonful three times a day in juice with meals.

5. Garlic, as previously mentioned, actively encourages the growth of benign flora in the colon and acts as an antiseptic, destroying unfriendly bacteria. Garlic is also one of the few herbs that not only kills intestinal parasites but also actively expels them.

6. Cascara sagrada bark, senna pods and/or leaves, and aloes are all rich in *emodin*. Emodin has a direct action on the smooth muscle of the large intestine, stimulating it and encouraging it to move. Aloes are generally twice as strong as cascara sagrada. The two best known are cape aloes and curacao aloes, and these are much more powerful than aloe vera. The juice of aloe vera or its gel are commonly available in health food shops and have much milder properties than either cape or curacao aloes in their whole form.

CORRECTIVE FORMULAS

The following formulas are designed to help proper bowel function and aid in elimination.

Intestinal Corrective Formula 1

This is a unique and unbeatable formula for treating bowel problems and is also helpful as part of a treatment for haemorrhoids. Its aim is to restore normal bowel function, not to create dependence. The combination of herbs in this formulation cleanses the liver and gall-bladder, starts the bile flowing, and stimulates peristalsis so that the layers of encrusted ancient mucus can gradually slough off as the bowel is rebuilt, resulting in the perfect assimilation of food. It also heals inflamed areas and relaxes areas of tension. It was originally developed by Dr Christopher, the world famous American herbalist.

- -

One part of: *red raspberry leaves*
barberry bark   *turkey rhubarb root*
cayenne pepper   *fennel*
goldenseal   *Two parts of:*
lobelia   *cascara sadgrada*

Buy all these herbs in powdered form and mix them well together by sieving. Then fill size 0 gelatin capsules with the mixture.

Begin by taking two capsules, three times a day with meals, or if you don't eat three times a day, take two capsules with every meal that you do eat. The aim is to achieve a bowel movement for every meal ingested. If you get diarrhoea, cut down the dosage. If you cannot get a movement then raise the dosage until you can.

- -

The dosage of this formulation produces very individual results and must be monitored and adjusted according to individual response. You will need to regulate the dose of this formula according to your own needs.

The bits of encrusted mucus that emerge over time may look very odd. You may see nuts and seeds that have been lodged in the colon for months or even years; traces of barium meal (if you have ever had one); bits of what may look like rubber tyre, tree bark or coloured Vaseline jelly. Alternatively, bowel movements may emerge smelling particularly foul or may come out accompanied by a great deal of rumbling or flatulence. Don't be alarmed by any of this. **Do not taper off the formulation so much that you lose momentum and the continuity of this wonderful elimination**.

This formulation must, of course, be coupled with correct diet, attitude adjustments, and a good exercise programme in order to be effective. You will simply be wasting your efforts if you neglect any of these facets of the programme. As the colon cleanses, heals and rebuilds itself, you will be able to taper off and finally finish the formulation altogether.

Intestinal Corrective Formula 2

This is Richard Schulze's formulation. He is Principal of the College of Herbs and Natural Healing in the UK, and an internationally recognised authority on herbal medicine.

This brilliant stimulating tonic is both cleansing and healing to all parts of the gastro-intestinal system. It disinfects, halts putrefaction, stimulates peristalsis, soothes and heals the mucous membrane lining of the digestive tract, relieves gas and cramps, improves digestion, increases the flow of bile which is cleansing to the gall-bladder, bile ducts and liver, promotes healthy intestinal flora, acts as an antibacterial, anti-viral, anti-fungal, destroys intestinal parasites and increases gastro-intestinal circulation. It is three or four times stronger than the Intestinal Corrective Formula 1.

Two parts: *cape aloes*
senna leaves and pods   *barberry root*
cascara sagrada   *ginger root*
One part: *cayenne*
curaco aloes   *garlic*

Buy all these herbs in powdered form and mix well together by sieving them. Then fill size 0 gelatin capsules.

Begin with one capsule before each meal and increase the dose by one capsule every other day until the desired number of bowel movements is reached. If you are taking more than one capsule at a time be sure to space them out.

Contra indication: Do not use during pregnancy.

Intestinal Corrective Formula 3

This soothing and cleansing formula is to be used alongside Intestinal Corrective Formula 1 and 2. It is designed, again by Richard Schulze, to be a strong purifier to the intestinal tract. It will draw out old, hardened faecal debris from the wall of the colon. It will also draw out toxins, poisons, heavy metal such as mercury and lead as well as radioactive elements like Strontium 90. The charcoal in formula 3 has the ability to draw out 2,000 different kinds of chemical drugs from the bowel and through the bowel wall from the blood and lymphatic systems. Its natural mucilaginous properties make it an excellent remedy for inflammation of the stomach and intestines. This property is also valuable for softening hardened, dried faecal matter for easy removal.

Two parts: *licorice root*
psyllium seeds   *carob pod, powdered*
ground flax seeds   *slippery elm bark*
charcoal, powdered   *bentonite clay*
One part: *fruit pectin*

Mix well. Dosage is one rounded teaspoonful two to five times daily. Mix in a blender with 4 to 6 fl oz of juice diluted half and half with water. It is essential to drink an additional 16 fl oz of any type of liquid after every dose of this formulation.

CHAPTER 5:

SELF MONITORING: GENITO-URINARY HEALTH AND BREAST HEALTH

———

• VAGINAL HEALTH •

More women seek medical attention for vaginal infections than for any other problems. Yet even today, many liberated women have no idea what a healthy vagina should look, smell, feel or taste like. A lot of women on the pill do not appreciate what normal vaginal secretions are like, simply because the pill tends to distort or diminish them. Droplets of fluid form on the vaginal walls and mix with the dead and sloughed off cells giving the secretions a white, milky appearance. The cervical canal secretes a thicker mucus, either clear or white, and this too flows into the vagina. Vaginal secretions are usually slightly acid and cervical secretions are slightly acidic when white, non-fertile mucus is being secreted, but become alkaline when secretions are clear and fertile. How much a woman secretes is variable. Women on the pill have very little secretion at any time of the month but those using natural contraceptive methods can often have a lot of secretion at ovulation time.

It generally used to be the case that only diabetics and pregnant women experienced repeated vaginal infections. But nowadays, my own observations among my patients suggest that these have become major problems for many women. Vaginitis, as these infections are collectively called, causes a vaginal discharge of some sort, pain, itching, pain on intercourse and sometimes painful urination. The organisms that cause the trouble are the normal residents of the vaginal environment but they have somehow become out of balance. They include bacteria and yeasts that usually shelter happily in the secretions that coat the vaginal walls. Sometimes intercourse, the simple friction of the penis against the vaginal wall, is enough to rub the cells from the wall in the same way that external skin is rubbed off by friction, allowing bacteria to penetrate the deeper layers where they may grow unchecked. Other vaginal irritants include:
- tight clothing
- synthetic fibres
- various contraceptive aids including diaphragms

- condoms and IUD strings
- tampons, which not only stop the free drainage of vaginal fluids but are also treated with chemicals
- spermicidal creams
- deodorant sprays
- bubble baths and soap
- detergents, if not rinsed out of underwear thoroughly
- vibrators
- various chemical drugs, especially antibiotics
- synthetic douche solutions.

Naturally stress will influence vaginal health as it does every other part of the body and a prolapsed colon, poor pelvic muscle tone or poor diet can also result in vaginitis.

HYGIENE

Any itching, irritating or smelly discharge should immediately be checked professionally – this includes an itchy vulva which may be the result of infection in the anal area. Skin conditions such as psoriasis can affect the vulva, as can diabetes. Atrophic dermatoses, where the vulval skin becomes thin in parts and thickened and lumpy in others, needs professional help from a medical herbalist, but most vulval irritations are simply dealt with. Always remember to keep the vulval area clean and as dry as possible. Wash daily with plain water or, if you insist, use a little natural soap. Wipe your bottom from front to back and wear only cotton or silk underwear. When I found that talcum powder might be one of the contributive factors to cancer of the ovaries I stopped using it immediately and now on the rare occasions I need any powder in the vulval area I use a little corn starch – this is a good tip for powdering babies' bottoms too.

FEMININE SPRAYS

Please avoid any kind of so-called feminine spray. Your vagina, if healthy, is beautifully and brilliantly designed to look after itself without much conscious help. The inside of the vagina is lined with flattened mucus epithelial cells, some thirty deep, that are continually shed rather like skin cells and these are decomposed by harmless resident bacteria producing lactic acid which protects the vagina against harmful bacteria. A study of 348 women showed that those who use deodorant sprays and douches had a higher instance of vulvovaginitis (inflammation of the vagina and the vulva) than non-users.

DOUCHES

While these are the oldest solution to vaginal infections they should never be used on a healthy vagina and never during pregnancy. When taking a douche (see page 44) the tip of the appliance should be inserted all the way into the vagina so that it actually touches the cervix. The vaginal opening should then be well sealed with the hand so that the douche solution fills, stretches and cleans every part of the vagina. A douching kit, after use, needs to be cleaned with hot running water and thoroughly dried.

VAGINAL SECRETIONS

The odour and appearance of a discharge are important clues in identifying any kind of infection. A healthy woman's vulval odour usually smells pleasant and somewhat musky while a bacterial infection will often smell very fetid, and a parasitic infection sour or fishy. A fungal infection will smell of yeast and is usually heavy, thick, curdy and white, or occasionally tinged with grey or green. Bacterial infections tend to be brownish and runny. It is possible to have more than one infection at a time. Women's individual vaginal secretions vary but if any kind of infection is present they normally become more copious. Besides the vagina being red and swollen and tender the vulva and inner lips can become swollen and irritated, and itching can be intense.

> *When treating any kind of vaginal infection it is essential to get an accurate diagnosis from a professional. This is particularly important if you suspect you have one of the major sexually transmitted diseases, such as syphilis or gonorrhoea. These diseases are not suitable for home treatment so are not covered in this book.*

LEUCORRHOEA

This is the medical term for any whitish discharge from the vagina. Remember that what is normal for one woman might be abnormal for another. Simply look for a change from your usual patterns as changes point to possible trouble especially if there is also itching and pain. If you are worried, do a three-day vegetable juice fast and include plenty of hot potassium broth (see p. 15). Every hour drink half a cup of the following decoction.

Two parts:	dandelion
blue flag	echinacea
sage	goldenseal
One part:	parsley root

Douche with a teaspoonful of goldenseal tincture in two litres of warm water or, if you are growing your own wheat grass, a few tablespoonfuls of the juice in two litres of water.

If mild vaginitis is a constant problem, take a nightly sitz bath in hot water in which you have dissolved half a cup of table salt. Insert your finger into the vagina and let the salty water flow into the vaginal canal. The saline solution will help to reduce the population of any invading or excessive organisms so shoring your body's defences.

THRUSH (CANDIDA ALBICANS – ALSO KNOWN AS MONILIASIS AND CANDIDIASIS)

The fungus Candida albicans only produces problems when your body is out of balance, which allows it to multiply and change its forms. It loves moist, warm environments and the symptoms include intense itchiness, especially at night, soreness and a thick white discharge. It is very common in pregnancy, in women on the pill, in women taking antibiotics and for those engaging in active sex, because it lives under the foreskin of the penis, and can be transmitted during love making. The pill encourages a sweeter vaginal environment which in turn encourages fungal growth. (Also read the section on Candida albicans [see page 173].

Follow the systemic treatment recommended on page 174 and, in addition, take forty drops of echinacea tincture every hour while awake. Douche morning and evening with either garlic water or black walnut. To make the garlic water simply crush two cloves of fresh garlic into two litres of warm water and allow to stand for twenty minutes before straining out the garlic. To make black walnut douche, add two teaspoonfuls of black walnut tincture to two litres of warm water.

If the itching is simply unbearable make a poultice of slippery elm and gold-enseal, adding a touch of cider vinegar when mixing, and spread this thick paste over the vulva and labia, securing it in position with a sanitary towel. After washing pat dry with a clean towel and wipe the whole area with olive oil which will prevent the yeast from proliferating. Remember to get your partner checked out too just in case you are passing the infection back and forth.

TRICHOMONAS

Trichomonas vaginitis (abbreviated to trich) is a one-celled parasite usually transmitted by sexual contact as it thrives under the foreskin of a penis in the male urethra and in the prostate gland. Most of the partners of women suffering from trich will be infected by it too. Lesbians transmit it very rarely. Very occasionally it can be caught from moist objects such as towels, flannels and toilet seats. The infection is occasionally manifested by burning, and sexual intercourse can be very sore.

The discharge produced is frothy, smelly and can be green, white or brownish while the vulva is reddened and mildly swollen. It has a tendency to recur the week after menstruation so douching for the whole week during this time is particularly helpful. Use two litres of garlic water in which a further teaspoonful of tincture of myrrh has been diluted. Men need to wash under their foreskin with this solution and wear a condom when making love for at least three months after the initial diagnosis.

The simplest, easiest and most successful treatment for trich is inserting a clove of raw garlic as high up into the vaginal canal as possible nightly. If you are worried about not being able to retrieve it wrap the clove in a piece of gauze 12 inches (30 cm) long and 1 inch (2.5 cm) wide. Fold this in half and twist it just below the clove making a small tampon with a long tail and then dip the clove end in olive oil and insert. Insert a clove of garlic morning and evening, taking the first clove out before putting the second clove in, so the first clove is left in all day and the second clove is left in all night. The garlic clove needs to be peeled before it is inserted and it should be gently bruised slightly between the fingers before doing so.

CHLAMYDIA TRACHOMATIS

Chlamydia attacks the cervix, the fallopian tubes, the liver and sometimes the eyes. The problem with chlamydia is that in women there are usually no symptoms at all. A woman may detect a vaginal discharge ranging from thin and white to copious green or yellow, she may have vulval and vaginal soreness, sexual intercourse might be painful and very occasionally urination may be painful or frequent. Men will get a sore on the urethra one or two weeks after contact making it painful to urinate, as well as a discharge from the penis and sometimes inflammation of the joints.

It is essential that both partners are treated because in women untreated chlamydia can cause chronic pelvic inflammatory disease and consequent infertility. When treating this I normally place a patient on a programme of high and frequent doses of antibiotic herbs, particularly echinacea, goldenseal and garlic. You should not attempt to treat Chlamydia without seeking professional help.

If you want to get pregnant I recommend that you have a genital swab taken for chlamydia. If it is positive your doctor will be able to advise the best course of action.

NON-SPECIFIC VAGINITIS

This is a general term which is used when the agent responsible for causing the trouble cannot be firmly identified. Bacterial infections can be caused by the overgrowth of bacteria which travel from an infection in the urinary tract or the intestinal tract to the vagina, and they can be also be passed on during love making, if your partner has a urethral infection, or after anal intercourse if the penis is not washed before vaginal insertion. The multiplication of bacteria will cause pain, itching and runny, foul smelling, usually brown discharge. Take forty drops of equal combinations of echinacea and goldenseal every three hours while awake, eat three to six cloves of raw garlic daily, and douche with any of the following combinations:

One tablespoonful of apple cider vinegar and one clove of garlic crushed into two litres of water. Remove the garlic after macerating it in the water for twenty minutes. Use one to two times a day for three to five days.

A cool infusion of plantain leaves. Douche with two litres of this mixture strained, twice a day for two weeks.

A strained and cooled infusion of equal parts of chamomile, sage, goldenseal and comfrey. Use one to two times a day for three to five days adding a tablespoonful of apple cider vinegar to two litres of this mixture before douching each time.

Usually douching once or at most twice per day for three or four days is enough to clear an infection completely. If it does not please seek professional help.

TOXIC SHOCK SYNDROME

The membranes of the vagina are extremely absorbent and very sensitive indeed to toxic substances. Many woman, quite understandably, feel that tampons are a godsend and use them throughout every period without realising the substances they contain. If incorrectly used, tampons are capable of causing drying, micro-ulceration and ulceration of the vaginal membranes. This is because tampons are capable of absorbing sixty-five per cent of menstrual blood and thirty-five per cent of genital secretions. It is also possible for strands of their fibrous material to become embedded in the vaginal membrane.

Symptoms

Tampons have also been unequivocally linked with toxic shock syndrome. A bacterium called Staphylococcus aureus has been associated with toxic shock syndrome and this bacteria produces TSS-Toxin 1, but considerable uncertainty is still present about the exact cause of this disease. However, it has been established that for every gram in tampon absorbency the risk of toxic shock syndrome increases by thirty-seven per cent. While toxic shock syndrome is extremely rare, affecting perhaps only three in 100,000 women, it can be fatal. Symptoms include a sudden high temperature, a drop in blood pressure, a sunburn-like rash followed one or two weeks later by skin peeling, especially on the hands and feet. Other symptoms may include nausea, vomiting or diarrhoea, muscle aches, bloodshot eyes or a sore throat, kidney problems, decreased liver function, lowered number of blood platelets, dizziness, disorientation and organ damage.

There is some suggestion that the applicator may make tiny cuts or abrasions in the vaginal wall on insertion, but whatever the cause of toxic shock syndrome I would strongly recommend that **you do not use tampons**, especially in view of some of the unnatural material they contain.

What are tampons made of?

In the past tampons were made with one hundred per cent artificial fibres such as polyacrylate, but these have now been withdrawn from the market and a mixture of cotton and rayon is used instead. Rayon is made from woodpulp derived cellulose which is occasionally subject to contamination with dioxins. The cotton used is often sprayed with pesticides. In Sweden there is now concern that the dioxins used as part of the bleaching process of the cotton may contribute towards cancer of the uterus.

There is no legal obligation in Britain reveal the chemical contents of tampons but you can safely assume that most will contain some or all of the following substances:

- cotton
- fibres of rayon
- polyacrylates and polyester
- polyvinyl alcohols and ethers
- phenol derived from coal tar
- carboxymethyl cellulose.

SANITARY TOWELS

As with tampons, there is little legal regulation on the manufacture of sanitary towels. Neither tampons nor sanitary towels are sterilised because to sterilise them would hinder absorbency, or so the industry says. Women in the Third World do particularly badly because sanitary towels there have occasionally been found to contain high levels of bacteria and fungi as well as additions such as fishing hooks, needles, cockroach eggs and rat droppings. The material of which sanitary towels are made is exposed to organochlorines and dioxins at the woodpulping and bleaching stages of manufacture, as well as other chemical additives.

The natural option

However, it is now possible to buy unbleached sanitary towels (see Resources Directory) and some women go further than this and use natural sponges or sanitary towels made of unbleached cotton. If you do opt for a sponge, steaming it or letting it sit in very hot water with a generous dash of apple cider vinegar is the way to clean it. Boiling tends to destroy it.

Disposal

There is another factor here which needs to be borne in mind. Seventy-five per cent of blocked drains are caused by sanitary products. One of the most fundamental laws of ecology is that everything must go somewhere and of course used sanitary towels and tampons are flushed into the sea via our sewage systems. Plastic applicators are becoming one of the largest plastic pollution problems in the seas.

They are eaten by all sorts of marine life including turtles, whales, fish, seals and sea birds, causing their death. Two million sea birds and 100,000 marine mammals die as the direct result of eating or being caught up in plastic. Far better to wrap your sanitary wear up and to dispose of it in the trash until you are in a position to burn it.

GENITAL WARTS

These are caused by the human papilloma virus (HPV) and are spread by sexual contact. Both men and woman can have them. HPV gravitates towards warm, moist areas in the vagina, round the anus and labia and on the cervix. The warts can be tiny or large cauliflower-like growths. They are extremely contagious. Even underwear can carry the virus and cause the return of warts, so wear fresh underwear every day. If your partner has warts on his hands ensure that he does not give you any genital stimulation until they are cleared up.

Genital warts, as with warts on any other part of the body, have a mysterious life of their own and can clear up spontaneously, particularly immediately after pregnancy. Naturopathically the cause of warts is no different from any other viral, bacterial or parasitic infection, but is simply due to the lowered vitality and lack of resistance on the part of the host: Warts are more frequently found in areas exposed to trauma or repeated friction and can be made more painful by friction during sexual activity.

Treatment

I have used castor oil poultices over the genital area on patients with this problem with a great deal of success. Black walnut tincture taken internally is also very helpful; the normal dose would be fifteen drops three times a day. I would also recommend plenty of raw garlic. Raw garlic can also be used as a poultice over the wart but must be applied extremely accurately as it will burn healthy tissue. I would recommend painting around the area with a cotton swab liberally soaked in olive oil before a slice of garlic is applied and fixed with a small piece of butterfly tape. A garlic poultice is best suited to smooth areas and you do need to persist for four to six weeks to see good results. Hypnosis has also been found to be remarkably effective for warts.

PUBIC LICE (CRABS)

These are like head lice but they infest pubic hair. They are generally caught through having sexual intercourse with an infected partner but they can thrive anywhere on the body including the head, underarms, eye brows and eye lashes. In some parts of the world they carry typhus, but generally in the Western world they are more annoying than dangerous. The first sign of infection is itching in the area where they have settled. The eggs take from seven to nine days to hatch and each crab lays about three eggs a day. The crabs themselves are minute and extremely difficult to see. The eggs show up more clearly as small brown specks at the base of the hair shaft.

Crabs are so easily transmitted an entire household can be infected by sharing the same couch or toilet. Simply sharing a bed with someone who has them often leads to infection. Crabs like to nest in sleeping bags and rugs. They cannot live longer than twenty-four hours without blood from people and the eggs can survive in clothing for up to a week, so if the bedding or clothing concerned is not washed or used for a week the eggs will die of their own volition.

For quick relief from the itching massage apple cider vinegar, garlic oil or black walnut tincture into the area. In addition drink half a cup three times a day of the following mixture and make a compress of it to apply over the affected area overnight.

Six ·parts: *cinnamon powder*
hyssop   *cloves powder*
One part: *lobelia*
walnut leaves or inner bark   *ginger*
Half a part:

HERPES

This is caused by the herpes simplex virus and both herpes simplex virus types can be responsible. HSV-1, the common cold sore virus, can cause an attack of genital herpes if it is transferred from cold sores on your partner's or your own lips. HSV-2 is usually transmitted sexually. Tests have shown that HSV-2 can live up to four hours on toilet seats.

The time from exposure to herpes until the time the blisters develop is between two and twelve days and the blisters are sometimes preceded by flu-like feelings and a low grade fever. In women they will appear on the mucous membranes of the lips, clitoral hood, vagina, anus or cervix and in men on the penis, scrotum and anus. The blisters are small, often break and weep and scab over and usually cause severe burning or itching. Sometimes lymph nodes located in the groin can become enlarged. The first bout of herpes is often the worst but it is common to have recurrences. Many women notice that herpes will flair up during menstruation or return when resistance is lowered due to illness, fatigue, sunburn or any other stress, or as the result of severe physical friction. While herpes can be merely annoying for some women, for others it can be debilitating.

Relief from Herpes

It is helpful to keep the sores as dry as possible and to wear loose-fitting cotton clothing. Warm garlic sitz baths are an excellent idea but it is important to dry the sores thoroughly after bathing. Some of my patients suggest using a hand-held hair dryer set on cool to dry any residual moisture. Ice-packs are also extremely helpful and if urination is painful, put a liberal layer of Vaseline over the blisters beforehand or sit in a bath of coolish water while urinating. Keep your diet as alkaline as possible and drink a couple of pints of potassium broth a day, avoiding alcohol while the attack lasts. Powdered goldenseal applied locally as a mini poultice is extremely effective as is the following combination of herbs.

Drink one cup of decocted oregan grape root tea three times a day. In each cup put fifteen drops of the following combinations of tinctured herbs: equal parts of goldenseal, garlic and skullcap or Echinacea complex.

Complications

A potentially serious complication arising from herpes is the risk of transmission of the virus from a woman to her baby at birth. If there are herpes blisters present at the time of birth the virus can be passed from the woman to the baby as it passes down the birth canal during delivery. This is particularly dangerous because the damage can be fatal and a caesarean birth is generally recommended.

BARTHOLIN CYSTS

The Bartholin glands secrete lubricating fluid around the opening of the vagina. In good health they cannot be felt and their openings are barely seen, but when they are infected they can swell up from their normal bean size to the size of a walnut and become extremely painful. Pain and swelling of the vulva may indicate infection of one or both of these small glands which lie just outside the opening of the vagina. Sometimes walking is painful since pelvic motion causes friction in the area of the gland and you may actually feel as if there is a stone in your vulva or a little bit of misplaced bone because the lump can be so hard. A hot compress of goldenseal powder is extremely helpful, as are sitz baths taken as hot as you can manage. Take a sitz bath morning and evening and after doing so refresh the compress. Also eat plenty of raw garlic and take two size 0 capsules of goldenseal every four hours until the infection has drained or passed completely and the pain or swelling has gone.

● WOMB CARE ●

FIBROIDS

A very large number of women live with fibroids in their uteruses, have children and experience minimum inconvenience. Fibroids are simply non-malignant growths of smooth muscle and fibrous connective tissue which can range from the size of a pea to the size of a grapefruit. Thirty per cent of all women over thirty are estimated to have these benign tumours. Starting inside the uterus, many fibroids can often occur simultaneously on the uterine wall or on the outer surface of the uterus. Sometimes they can grow out from the uterus on a stalk and if the stalk twists the blood supply can be cut off causing pain or vaginal discharge. They can cause very heavy uterine bleeding and discharge and heavy painful periods. Some miscarriages occur because the fibroids fill the cavity and irritate the uterine lining. If very large fibroids can press against the bladder causing frequent urination, or against the colon interfering with normal bowel movements, or against nerve endings causing pain and an overall feeling of fullness in the abdomen. Fibroid growth is stimulated by hormones, particularly oestrogen, and with each menstruation fibroids can grow a little larger. The pill can accelerate their growth and during pregnancy because hormone levels are higher, fibroids grow faster. Once the menopause arrives they can often shrink and disappear.

Removal of the fibroids in a procedure called myomectomy is offered to women who want to get pregnant but can't as a result of the fibroids. Cutting the uterus results in scar tissue which in rare cases inhibits dilation of the cervix during labour. However, I know women who have had successful vaginal births after uterine surgery.

I have also worked very successfully with this problem herbally but the treatment is long and requires persistence and dedication. Consult a medical herbalist if you are interested in following this route.

VAGINAL BOLUS

A bolus is a way of administering herbs vaginally other than on a tampon or by douching. Boluses are made with healing herbs that draw out toxins and poisons so making the malfunctioning area healthy. They spread their herbal influence widely from the vagina or bowel through the entire urinary and genital organs.

Mix up equal parts of squawvine, slippery elm, yellow dock, comfrey, marshmallow, chickweed, goldenseal and mullein, all in finely powdered form and then melt down enough coconut butter to mix in well with the powders so that the whole mass has the texure of pastry. Now roll it between the hands until you have a pencil-like bolus as thick as your thumb and about one inch long. Round off the ends gently with your fingers and harden the boluses on a greased baking sheet in the fridge. Insert one of these boluses for six nights a week before bed. Protect your underwear with a sanitary towel and fast on the seventh day. Overnight the coconut butter will melt leaving only the herbs which are easy to douche out.

The following morning lie on your slant board (see Appendix 3) and inject half a cup of the following mixture with your douche applicator.

Six parts: mullein
comfrey   marshmallow
oak bark   walnut
Four parts: One part:
yellow dock   lobelia
Three parts:

Make as a decoction (see p. 40) and strain well before use. Hold this mixture in the vagina as long as possible before voiding. While doing so knead and massage the abdominal area, also doing your slant board exercises (see Appendix 3) so that the herbal tea can be assimilated by the body.

Using this treatment six days on and one day off, I have helped women with fibroids. Certainly, upon repeated physical examination they become smaller and smaller and eventually disappear altogether.

POLYPS

Polyps are growths that form along the endocervical canal and protrude from the inside of the uterus or on the face of the cervix. They are soft red tube-like growths which are benign and can cause a discharge and possible bleeding when irritated. I have had some success helping women with these using the following formulation:

Equal parts: false unicorn root
blessed thistle   ginger
red raspberry   licorice
cayenne pepper   uva ursi
goldenseal   squawvine
cramp bark

All the herbs should be powdered. Take two size O capsules morning and evening. Or try Nature's Way Femaprin. Be persistent for six months with either of these treatments and if bleeding becomes heavier seek professional help.

ENDOMETRIOSIS

A growing number of women are being diagnosed with endometriosis and it is the second most common gynaecological disorder that requires hospital treatment.

Endometriosis occurs when tissue like that in the lining of the womb is found in other parts of the body including the ovaries, fallopian tubes and peritoneum. Deposits have been found all over the body including the lungs and the eyes. These deposits bleed during every menstrual period – they behave just as if they are in the womb lining. The bleeding causes inflammation and adhesions can form, which may make organs stick to one another.

Menstruation

Menstruation can be very painful for some women with endometriosis and the inflammation can give *constant* discomfort, not just at period times. It can make intercourse very uncomfortable and symptoms may also include bloating, heavy or erratic bleeding, constipation or diarrhoea and unsurprisingly, extreme fatigue and depression. Symptoms can be relatively painful for women who show very little endometrial tissue.

Research

Researchers are still investigating the cause(s) of endometriosis. Interesting new research done by the United States Endometriosis Protection Agency suggests a close link between dioxin levels in the body and the severity and incidents of endometriosis. An experiment carried out on rhesus monkeys exposed to TCDD, the most toxic dioxin, found that the incident of endometriosis was directly correlated with dioxin exposure. Further research showed the severity of disease was dependent upon the dose administered.

If this is the case it is doubly important that women do not use sanitary towels or tampons but find some other alternative (see page 81). As dioxins are airborne, falling on grass and plants eaten by farmed animals, it is essential to cut out all dairy produce from the diet.

Drugs

Endometriosis appears mainly in women between the ages of thirty and forty-five and pregnancy is believed to protect a woman from endometriosis which usually begins to disappear after the menopause. One of the reasons for this is that endometriosis may be hormonally linked to an over-production of oestrogen, and production of oestrogen ceases after the menopause.

Indeed HRT, in which oestrogen is released into the bloodstream of post-menopausal women, has been known to reactivate symptoms.

Current drug therapy for endometriosis aims to suppress ovulation, inducing a state like pregnancy or the menopause. Danazol which is one of the most commonly used drugs for endometriosis and another drug gestrinone both induce a post-menopausal state. They are both androgens, similar to male reproductive hormones. Side-effects of their use can include greasy skin, hirsutism (hairiness), voice changes which are non-reversible and acne.

Surgeons can remove the lining of the womb to stop heavy bleeding using a variety of techniques, including laser. However, it is known to be a risky procedure.

Herbal treatments

I have had considerable success working with women with endometriosis but persistence and discipline is necessary. I use the female corrective on page 114 and the same treatment as for fibroids on page 85. If there is pain a nervine sedative on page 158 can be administered. Alternatively, drink a decoction of equal parts of valerian and cramp bark tea, if necessary a cup every half hour. Hot and cold sitz baths are also extremely helpful. Add ten drops of cypress oil to the hot water.

Far from the pill protecting against endometriosis, as is sometimes claimed, it may actually be responsible for some cases of it.

PELVIC INFLAMMATORY DISEASE

Pelvic inflammatory disease (PID) is also known as salpingitis (inflammation of the fallopian tubes), and salpingo-oophoritis (inflammation of the ovaries and fallopian tubes). Do not attempt to self-treat PID without first taking professional advice.

Pelvic inflammatory disease is a generalised term used to describe any kind of acute or chronic infection affecting the pelvic area. Acute PID manifests with a high temperature and pelvic pain with signs of genital infection. Chronic PID can be the cumulative result of several past infections, especially chlamydia and gonorrhoea. Any infection will make the fallopian tubes and ovaries more vulnerable. If untreated, the inflammation will leave you with heavy painful periods and back-ache. Intercourse is often painful and may trigger bleeding. You may notice unusual vaginal discharges, have problems urinating and have a generally swollen and uncomfortable abdomen. Feeling ill and run down all the time becomes the norm. If not treated promptly, the final result may be infertility.

Cause of infection

Our gynaecological system, like every other part of the body, is designed to be self-protecting. The fallopian tubes and ovaries are anatomically open to the outside world and all its foreign infective agents via the uterus and vagina. Happily they are protected by their own built-in self-defence mechanisms and barriers. The vagina is generally acidic except during menstruation; this stops bacteria from flourishing. The thick mucus plug of the cervix is a further mechanical barrier to bacterial invasion and the hair-like cilia in the uterus and fallopian tubes waft any bacteria downwards towards the cervix and vagina, acting in much the same way as they do in the nose. During menstruation the cervical mucus plug is not effective and the vagina changes to alkaline, but normally the infection is held at bay by a healthy menstrual flow. After pregnancy these self-defences are reduced. Infection may be introduced during the delivery as a result of tissue trauma. After childbirth there is prolonged vaginal discharge which can last for two to six weeks so the possibility of an ascending infection becomes greater. Most cases of salpingitis due to ascending infection follow birth or a botched abortion. Old-fashioned IUDs were sometimes the cause of ascending infections due to the introduction of bacteria on insertion or to mechanical irritation and congestion which creates a good environment for bacterial growth. Poor circulation round the ovaries and fallopian tubes of both blood and lymph can be the result of constipation, diverticulitis or appendicitis or it may be the result of lack of exercise, a poor diet or psychological trauma.

Treatment

> *I emphasise again it is very important to catch any pelvic infection early and treat it promptly.*

However, a low-grade infection may produce symptoms which simply mimic pain or cramping with a period and so remain undetected. I have assisted women to heal themselves of both acute and chronic PID with a great deal of success. Obviously the chronic version requires much dedication and persistence as well as considerable courage as the pain can often be extreme. Women with chronic PID will often come to me heavily battered with long courses of antibiotics, which is the only thing the medical profession have to offer besides surgical intervention.

During acute attacks I always recommend fasting on apple or carrot juice with plenty of potassium broth for as long as the attack lasts, ensuring the colon is functioning extremely well. Hot and ice-cold abdominal packs applied alternatively as long as the pain lasts also help. Change these every two to three minutes and keep the rest of the body warm while applying them. If heat appears to be making the inflammation more painful apply only cold compresses every twenty minutes with ten minute breaks in between until the pain is calmed.

Alternating morning and evening hot and cold sitz baths with lavender oil added is extremely helpful. Massage ten drops of lavender oil diluted in a teaspoonful of almond oil into the lower back and abdomen daily. Take two female corrective (see page 114) morning and evening and during the course of an attack take very high doses of echinacea (360 drops during the course of the day in all). Fasting should be done on a regular basis for chronic PID and I generally recommend one regular day every week. All forms of hydrotherapy, including Turkish baths, cold plunges, saunas and cold showers, help to get the general circulation moving and should be taken at least twice per week. Regular skin brushing morning and evening helps. Between fasts, the diet should be vegan. There are some yogic positions which are particularly helpful for PID and a qualified yoga teacher will show you these.

CERVICAL EROSION

Doctors often refer to the redness of the cervix as cervical erosion and many women find this term frightening because it conjures up a picture of the cervix being eaten away like earth after heavy rainfall. It is important to understand that many women have red cervixes most of the time and that as this is part of their natural make-up there is absolutely nothing wrong with them. However, redness in conjunction with:

- a heavy white or yellow discharge;
- spotting or bleeding from the inflamed area of the cervix;
- pain during sexual intercourse or burning during urination;
- lower back pain accompanied by a slight fever

may all indicate infection and do need attention.

THE PAP SMEAR TEST

The pap smear test is used to identify women who may be at risk of developing cervical cancer. It can also detect the established condition. I'm not sold on this kind of screening for reasons discussed below. The likelihood of developing cervical cancer increases with the number of sexual partners and smoking. The risk is also influenced by whether you began your sex life early or have ever had any sexually transmitted disease. If you are at risk a pap smear test carried out under the right conditions and meticulously examined by an experienced technician may be advisable.

The test

During a smear test an open speculum is used to expose the cervix and vaginal walls. Cells from the face of the cervix are taken with a wooden spatula. Cells from the vaginal wall are also taken. These samples are then smeared onto a microscope slide and set with a fixative. The only thing you will feel is mild pressure.

The slide is then stained with a series of dyes and studied under a microscope for abnormal cell growth that could be pre-cancerous or cancerous, and for bacteria that cause vaginal infections. Laboratory technicians need to be skilled and alert as interpretations can vary wildly depending upon who is looking at the slide. Indeed it is possible to get a different interpretation from the same person looking at the same slide on separate occasions. If you are told you have a suspicious smear please seek a second opinion. It is vital to realise that cervical cancer is a very slow-developing disease giving a woman plenty of time to consult other medical opinions and consider what, if any, treatment is appropriate. Pre-cancerous changes do not inevitably lead to cancer. I had an abnormal smear test myself after a divorce, but I cleared it up within three months by simply taking an excellent diet with lots of raw foods and plenty of carrot juice, with alternate hot and cold sitz baths morning and evening to stimulate my circulation.

OVARIAN CYSTS

These are quite common. Often there are no symptoms, but there can be a little swelling in the lower abdomen, pain during sexual intercourse or irregularities in the menstrual cycle. Occasionally there may be discomfort or difficulty in having a bowel movement and urinary retention.

> **It is essential to get a proper and accurate diagnosis as a swollen or painful ovary can denote other illnesses.**

One ovary with several ovarian cysts is described as a *polycystic ovary*.

Treatment

If you have ovarian cysts, try taking a daily liver flush and follow the programme outlined on pp 63–4.

Take two size 00 capsules of change ease morning and evening. The formula consists of equal parts of powdered blessed thistle, false unicorn, true unicorn, licorice, sage, squawvine, Siberian ginseng and black cohosh. Or use Higher Nature's pre-mens prevention. Include plenty of purple dulse in your diet to regulate your thyroid.

Take alternate hot and cold sitz baths morning and evening. Skin brushing gently over your abdomen will help to improve circulation and providing you are not too tender, general skin brushing will also help.

If the ovarian cyst is causing acute abdominal pain, nausea or fever, this is an emergency situation. Seek immediate medical help. A cyst can haemmorrhage or rupture causing peritonitis. I had an ovarian cyst removed by surgery when I was 22. Having this type of surgery does not mean you lose the use of your ovary. It remains functional afterwards. Any subsequent problems may be the result of scar tissue which can impede the lymph and blood flow to the area but this can be successfully treated with moxa (this is the burning of a moxa stick over a specific point. Small wooden cones – usually artemsia – are burnt until they almost reach the skin. The process is similar to acupuncture but, as the herbs warm the skin, the effect is more gentle and comforting) and acupuncture by a qualified acupuncturist.

PROLAPSE

A uterine prolapse is a condition in which your uterus falls out of its proper place. It happens when the ligaments that support the uterus or the muscle supporting the pelvic floor has stretched. A vaginal prolapse, which is more common, is a condition where the walls of the vagina become weak allowing either the bladder or rectum or both to push into them. If the front of the vagina is weak the bladder bulges down and this can give you trouble when urinating and can cause incontinence. If the back wall is weak then the rectum bulges forward occasionally causing trouble with bowel function (Rectecele). The vagina may not feel as tight as it used to be and there may be sexual difficulties if the cervix is low down in the vagina. While most women who have a prolapse have had children, occasionally teenagers who have not had any children complain of trouble. Losing oestrogen after the menopause makes internal ligaments less supple and strong so most women with prolapses are over fifty. Being overweight, taking very little exercise, suffering from constipation and having a chronic cough all add extra strain.

Exercise

Contrary to popular belief a traumatic vaginal delivery does **not** lead to vaginal or uterine prolapse. The factor that makes a big difference is how often you exercise. What type of exercise really does not matter. Yoga, keep fit classes, walking, jogging, swimming or dancing are all helpful. Any type of exercise improves perineal (pelvic floor) muscle function. Such exercise acts preventively but if the pelvic floor muscles are already sagging you will need to do 200 Kegal exercises daily. The object is to contract and relax the muscle in a controlled manner, almost as if you were clenching and unclenching your fist. The contraction is the one you would use if you were trying to stop the flow of urine. Hold the contraction for five seconds before relaxing and then repeat four more times. The disadvantage of these exercises is that for them to be truly effective they have to be practised forty times a day which means 200 contractions in all.

For those women who don't remember to do this, get bored, simply haven't got the time or can't find the right muscles to contract, which is surprisingly common, the alternative is to buy vaginal weights. These are not quite as effective because they don't allow the muscles to relax in between contractions as the Kegal exercises do, but nevertheless they are helpful. I've used them extensively in my own practice. They can be inserted for twenty minutes every night while standing and doing something else and once a weight is held in comfortably for twenty minutes you can graduate to a heavier weight. Buy your own set and keep them clean (see Resources Directory). Yoga postures that help include the plough, and any inverted exercise.

I have used the following formulation many times with great success for prolapses. It was pioneered by Dr Christopher.

- -

Assemble six parts of oak bark, four parts of yellow dock, three parts of walnut leaves or bark, three parts of mullen, six parts of comfrey leaf, one part of lobelia and three parts of marshmallow root. Cover with an appropriate amount of purified water (if one part equals one ounce, then the amount of water would be six and a half pints). Decoct, simmering the whole mixture down to half its amount. Strain the mixture and inject vaginally or rectally, using the appropriate syringe (rectal or vaginal) depending on where the prolapse is. Lie on the slant board while doing so and retain for as long as possible before voiding. While on the slant board, perform the exercises (see Appendix 3) as this will help the tea's assimilation. You may also drink a quarter of a cupful, three times a day, diluting it if you find the taste too strong.

- -

Acupuncture

Acupuncture can also be extremely helpful in the early stages of prolapse. Traditional Chinese medicine says that a prolapse is the result of the spleen's failure to 'raise' the central organs. In layman's terms, this means the spleen is supposed to ensure that the central organs (stomach, kidneys, intestines and uterus) are kept in their normal position within the body. If the spleen's function of raising the central organs is disturbed then prolapse of one of these organs may occur. I have not, however, found acupuncture to be helpful in the later stages of prolapse.

Aromatherapy

Aromatherapists recommend massaging the lower back and abdomen with a combination of rose oil (5 drops) and lemon oil (5 drops) diluted in almond oil, ten drops of essential oils to one teaspoonful of base oil.

• KIDNEY/BLADDER CARE •

CYSTITIS

Cystitis is a term for inflammation of the bladder and it is not usually serious although it can be exceedingly uncomfortable. When the kidneys become infected the condition is know as *pyelitis*. Common symptoms include pain and burning on urination, cloudy, sour smelling or bloody urination, backache, chills and quite high fevers, none of which are to be taken lightly because the pain, distress and complete disruption of a woman's daily life resulting from bouts of cystitis can result in lost jobs, misery at home and even broken relationships.

Cause

Cystitis is often the result of bruising or trauma of the urethra and bladder, generally as the result of vigorous sexual activity, including masturbation, which promotes the growth of any bacteria which can be present. Such bruising and trauma happens when a hand, penis or mouth produces enough pressure and friction on the urethra and bladder to cause reddening and inflammation of these sensitive organs. The penis can harbour bacteria from the inflamed cervix, the anus or from vaginal infections and deposit them near a woman's urethral opening. Pressure on the urinary tract from an over-full bladder or bowel, from a diaphragm, or from a prolapsed uterus or vagina, can increase the possibility of urinary tract infection. During pregnancy it is not uncommon for the foetus to rest against and even kick the bladder or urethra, particularly in the last three months.

Escherichia coli (E. coli) is the bacteria commonly responsible for cystitis. It grows particularly well in blood and in vaginal secretions containing yeast so it is important to check, particularly if you are subject to repeated bouts of cystitis, that you are not also infected with candida. Even if you have candida it is very common to have negative bacterial counts on testing. Chlamydia can also cause cystitis. Chemical foams, sprays and douches can irritate the uretheral opening and spermicidal jellies or cream as well as the latex in condoms can produce irritation affecting the urethral entrance. Women who are diabetic have glucose in their urine which enables E. coli bacteria to thrive. Obstructions in the urinary tract, like kidney stones, can cause irritation and provide a focus for a growth of bacteria. This is a very simple instruction but it is absolutely essential that you sit down completely on the toilet seat while emptying your bladder. If you perch over the seat there is a very real possibility that the bladder won't be entirely empty and the stagnant urine left can set off another attack of cystitis.

Psychological factors

In many instances I have been aware of psychological factors in repeated attacks of cystitis and never really understood why until I realised that stress and related moods of depression stimulate the production of hormones which cause body cells to retain water. Since fluid is retained by the body's cells urine output is reduced and the bladder is flushed out less often, creating a good environment for bacteria. Counselling can be very helpful in overcoming psychological problems.

Treating Cystitis

- Do not wear tights.
- Do not wear anything other than cotton or silk underwear, both of which should be loose fitting.
- Avoid bleaches and detergents when washing clothing that touches the skin. Avoid fabric coloured by chemical dyes.
- Do not wash with soap; use cold running water especially immediately after sexual intercourse or masturbation.
- Urinate frequently before and after sex. This helps to relieve pressure and reduces the likelihood of bacterial build up.
- Do not use tampons or sanitary towels. During a period use a sponge fitted internally to catch the blood (See p.81).
- Constipation and liver congestion both cause toxins to be recirculated throughout the body and burden the kidneys with excess work, so ensure that your bowel is working beautifully. Do a liver flush once a month and as a preventive measure a kidney flush (see pages 62 and 95).

- Wipe from front to back using non-bleached, non-scented toilet paper, or use a bidet after urinating or defecating.
- In the event of an acute attack take a hot sitz bath every hour if this is practical.
- Fast on unsweetened cranberry juice, potassium broth and parsley tea. Solgar makes a good cranberry juice tablet.
- Take with a half a cup of kidney tea (page 65).
- Use a warm compress of fennel oil, ten drops diluted in enough water to moisten the compress, over the bladder and wrap yourself up well, keeping the rest of the body warm.
- For seven to ten days after the condition has subsided, while it is clearing, stay on a vegan diet including plenty of raw garlic, carrot juice and fluids. During this time either continue with the kidney flush or take twenty drops four times a day of couch grass tincture in plenty of water.

In really difficult cases of cystitis I have found reflexology extremely helpful.

KIDNEY STONES

Ninety per cent of kidney stones are made of calcium oxalate, a salt derived from oxalic acid which binds calcium together. It is important that your practitioner knows exactly what kind of stone to treat. A twenty-four hour urine test will help to determine this. If the problem is one of too much uric acid, it will require different treatment from a problem when oxalate levels are high and magnesium low. Magnesium helps increase the solubility of oxalates in the urine and vitamin B6 helps to control the body's production of oxalate acid, increasing oxalate excretion. Both are vital in preventing calcium oxalate stones which account for the majority. If this is the case a diet rich in vitamin B6 and magnesium is recommended, together with the following kidney flush.

- -

Kidney Flush

Juice of one lemon and one lime
16 to 32 fl oz of distilled water (hot or cold, as desired)
pinch of cayenne pepper
maple syrup (a little) to taste (optional)

Fifteen minutes after this drink, consume two cups of kidney/bladder tea (see p. 65) with two teaspoonfuls of kidney/bladder tonic added. Consume two more cups of this tea with the tonic added twice more each day.

- -

Kidney/Bladder Tonic

Three parts: cornsilk
uva ursi leaves   horsetail
dandelion leaf and root   gravel root
Two parts: golden rod
juniper berries   burdock
One part:

Make a tincture (see p. 40). Or use Cornsilk complex.

Some diets, including strict macrobiotic diets which can cause the urine to become very concentrated, are predisposed to stone formation. But an average Western diet also predisposes to kidney stones, being far too high in phosphorus and too low in calcium. This particularly applies to meat and fizzy drinks. Too much protein in the diet puts further strain on the kidneys creating a high level of sulphur amino acids and an acidic environment. A diet high in salt inhibits renal calcium reabsorption leading to an overall calcium loss.

Diet

If the kidney stones are the result of a problem with uric acid go on a three-day fast of carrot or apple juice once every fortnight for six months and include plenty of potassium broth in the diet on a daily basis. Avoid foods which are high in purine, which includes most meat and fish as well as yeast and porridge oats.

With either type of stone increase fluid intake to as much as you can manage, especially potassium broth. Ensure your water is filtered by a process of reverse osmosis and cut salt in all its forms out of the diet entirely.

Treatment

In the event of an acute attack apply a hot mullein poultice over the entire kidney area down to the small of the back and leave it on for thirty minutes. During this time keep the poultice as hot as possible. If necessary replace it with a second one and keep alternating them. Hot sitz baths will also help urine flow but for chronic kidney stones alternate hot and cold sitz baths are better. Take any of the following teas on a daily basis to ensure stones continue to dissolve: gravel root, horsetail, parsley, yarrow, dosage one cup three to six times a day. Follow the kidney cleanse programme on pp. 64–5 at least once a month.

Increasingly, research has discovered that a number of prescribed drugs may be the major cause of stone formation. This includes drugs used to treat glaucoma, congenital heart failure, hypertension, gastritis and heartburn, some diuretics and those used to prevent the body from rejecting transplants. Laxative abuse can also bring on kidney stones.

• BREAST HEALTH •

A woman who does breast self-examination on a regular basis is more likely to detect a change than any doctor or health worker doing a sporadic examination, so it is essential that you learn to examine your own breasts and become familiar with them.

HOW TO EXAMINE YOURSELF

The best time to do breast examination is on the first day after the period has finished. If you are undergoing menopause or are post-menopausal choose a regular day every month.

- Strip to the waist and stand in front of a mirror.
- Look at your breasts with your hands by your sides, first from the front and then in profile. What you are looking for are any dimples, large blood vessels, puckered skin or change in the shape or size of either breast.
- Now lift your arms over your head and check again. While doing so check that there is no swelling in the armpit or above the breast in this position.
- Using the flat part of your hand feel one breast using a circular motion round the nipple, working from the outside in. Check for any lumps or thickening. It is easier to do this if your skin is wet or soapy so you might prefer to do this part of the examination in the bath or under a shower.
- Finally check the nipple for any discharge. It is not unusual to have a little crust but a heavy discharge that is brown, green or bloody needs urgent medical attention.

If you find anything unusual whilst performing your regular examination, consult your GP.

BREAST CYSTS

The self-examination just described has, over the years, proved to be a very effective way of discovering breast cysts. Cysts are fluid-filled pockets ranging from the size of a pin to the size of a walnut. Thirty per cent of all women develop breast cysts at some point during their years of menstruation. Cysts move easily when touched, are hard and round and feel a bit like a firm blister. I've noticed cysts are more common in women who are taking the pill or other hormonal drugs; and if women steer clear of HRT cysts usually disappear after the menopause.

Breast cysts are common and normally benign, nevertheless the medical profession chooses to label them with long names such as fibrocystic disease or chronic cystic mastitis. These names often cause unnecessary alarm. Apart from hormones in the pill, hormones in meat aggravate breast cysts, as do chemicals found in coffee, tea, cola drinks and chocolate. Cutting all these out has a very positive affect, as does taking food high in vitamin E, including wheatgerm oil and flaxseed oil (See Resources Directory.). I would recommend one and a half tablespoonfuls a day added to the diet. Plenty of purple dulse in the diet also helps to correct hormonal imbalance. Skin brushing followed by hot and cold showers is important to assist circulation (see p. 61).

BREAST INFECTIONS

If you notice a greyish, greenish or yellowish liquid discharging from the nipple and can produce more liquid by pressing the sides of the nipples together, you probably have a bacterial infection in the breast ducts. Occasionally nipples can ooze milk during hormonal changes or from breast stimulation. This does not indicate infection. The indications of an infection are tender breasts, particularly around the nipples, fever and tender swollen lymph glands under the arms.

Seek immediate medical attention if the breast discharge is green in colour as the infection may be pseudomonas which can be extremely serious.

Breast infections are actually quite rare but bacterial infections can occur if there is a tiny break in the skin covering the nipple or if the bacteria has worked its way into the small ducts on the nipple itself.

Except where the infection is pseudomonas, breast infections can by treated by fasting on juices for as long as the infection lasts and by taking herbal antibiotics. Take two size 0 capsules every thirty to sixty minutes depending on how acute the infection is. Compresses of equal parts of mullein and lobelia applied as hot as possible to the affected area also help. Eat plenty of raw garlic.

• GENERAL HEALTH ADVICE •

CHOOSING A PRACTITIONER

If you are in good health go for a regular health check-up to a qualified therapist who is known to you either by personal recommendation or because they have proven their excellence to you in the past by their empathy, efficiency and intelligence. I do appreciate how hard it is to find the right practitioner but by putting yourself in for what is in effect a regular 5,000 miles service you will be practising wise prevention. Preventive medicine is hardly practised at all in the West, whereas, in many parts of China a practitioner only receives payment when a patient is well; payment stops abruptly when the patient becomes ill. Certainly an approach that would revolutionise health care! The practitioner you have chosen should be delighted to see you as they will seldom get the chance to practise preventive medicine. Normally the people who consult me are extremely ill which makes for much more emotional distress and hard work on both sides as well as making the whole process more expensive.

Your ideal practitioner should be an experienced holistic one with a profound knowledge of natural therapy and a sound familiarity with the best of modern medicine. The other advantage of finding somebody you trust on a preventive basis is knowing they will be there for you in an emergency.

Your first pre-requisite should be reputation. Ask the people you value and trust and get a few names and addresses to choose from, investigating them all. Alternatively contact the European Herbal Alliance (see Resources Directory for address). Your second priority should be to query what qualification that practitioner has. Find out how long their training took, make sure they belong to a professional association, obtain the address and check them out. Avoid therapists whose training was obtained over a weekend, or series of weekends. They may not be in a position to tell you the difference between a migraine and a brain tumour. However, they could be invaluable in addition to your main therapist.

Ensure that your main therapist is comfortable about referring you to other experts. I am well aware that the therapies in which I am trained have their limitations and I have built up a network of other alternative practitioners to whom I can turn for help, advice, a second opinion or referrals. This is the true concept of wholistic health care. Ask your therapist about his or her attitude to conventional medicine, and make sure you are comfortable with their views.

Your fourth criteria should be experience. Someone in full-time practice will almost always be better than a part timer. Choose somebody who has been in practice for at least three years. If an early appointment is unavailable this is usually an excellent sign. Many practitioners, however good they are and however heavily booked they are, reserve a few hours each week for true emergencies.

Make sure your therapist is willing to outline the likely cost of treatment and that he or she has a reasonably consistent scale of charges.

Finally rely on your intuition. If there isn't an empathy between you and your practitioner forget it and go and find someone else. When I was younger and inexperienced I succeeded in hurting myself several times by taking on people I couldn't warm to. The results were always disastrous. In my opinion there has to be a heart connection to make any kind of healing possible.

REGULAR CHECK-UPS

Allopathic testing

I would like to be able to tell you that I believe in cervical smear checks, mammograms, ultrasound scans, X-rays, etc., but I have to say that I have doubts about nearly all the methods of diagnosis that the allopathic profession uses. Even such simple tests as high blood pressure checks are known to be inaccurate. For example, emotional changes can alter blood pressure and some patients are so frightened of what their doctor will discover about their health that they develop a condition known as 'white coat hypertension' as soon as they step through the surgery door. Blood pressure rises when it is taken by the doctor and returns to normal as soon as they leave. If you have any worries about your blood pressure ambulatory monitoring it is probably more advisable. This is where you are fitted up with a device to measure blood pressure over a twelve-hour period. However, a French study found that even this system didn't provide accurate enough information for doctors to decide whether to treat the condition and the WHO now recommends that ambulatory monitoring is best conducted with multiple readings over six months. Urine tests, cholesterol tests, the haemoccult test (which can indicate cancer in the colon) and breath tests for lung problems are known to be reliable if properly conducted. I always feel more confident if I go to a practitioner who is capable of conducting a good physical examination but who also has access to alternative means of diagnosis such as applied kinesiology, iridology, mineral analysis done through hair tests, tongue and pulse diagnosis and posture analysis.

Diagnostic methods

If in doubt, don't diagnose yourself. Even GPs may be only fifty per cent accurate with diagnosis without access to pathology laboratories. Too often allopathic practitioners are only concerned with a narrow bio-medical approach to the treatment of disease and this results in a fragmented treatment. If you choose holistic medicine the best way to start on your journey to real health is to seek a professional naturopathic or medical herbal opinion first. The time to begin doing it yourself is after you have found out what needs to be done. It saves a lot of time, worry and money. Many of the diagnostic methods your naturopath or medical herbalist will use are ancient and well established and some are accepted by the scientific community.

Iridology coupled with Vega testing is my chosen diagnostic method. Iridology is the process used to diagnose conditions which involves analysing the iris of the eye. It reveals the presence of tissue inflammation in the body, its location and the stage it has reached. It is also a good indicator of constitutional strength, genetic patterns and inherent weaknesses. Vega testing concerns the ultra-fine measurements of cell wall electrical activity from an acupuncture point on the hand or foot. Using a series of ampules containing anything from food to organ tissue, the practitioner can carry out a wide range of diagnostic tests, establishing whether a person has any intolerances to food, drugs or other materials. It can also detect the rate at which the body is affected by these and which organs are touched. It will also indicate vitamin deficiencies, tumours (and other cystic processes or infections), geopathic stress, psychic disorders, Yin Yang balance (body polarity), acid-alkaline balance and compatibility to a given medication. I am also trained in physical examination – although physical examination alone is far too inaccurate. Hair analysis, radiasthesia, tongue, pulse and ear diagnosis (which the Chinese have used for centuries), aura measuring and colour therapy come from the past and all show promise for future use. I have never felt the need to beg orthodox medics to recognise how valid my art is, both in philosophy and in practice. Alternative medicine is simply a direct continuation of the healing arts and understanding practised and developed for centuries.

• WHAT TO LOOK FOR: WARNING SIGNS •

Obvious symptoms of a body under pressure include frequent coughs, sore throats, colds or flus, pain or strain anywhere in the body, skin irritations or eruptions, discharges of any sort from any orifice in the body, frequent fungal, bacterial or viral infections, depression, anxiety, fatigue, insomnia, irritability, hyperactivity, rapid weight swings, weakness, lack of concentration and a predisposition to so-called allergies.

If you develop any of the following warning signs, consult a qualified practitioner. For signs and symptoms marked * see your GP.

GENERAL WARNING SIGNS

- Feeling excessively tired, anxious or depressed.
- Losing weight.*
- Persistent cough.*
- Coughing up blood or heavy mucus, especially green or yellow mucus.*
- Lumps in your abdomen.
- Pain in the upper or lower abdomen.*

REPRODUCTIVE SYSTEM

- Bleeding or spotting after sexual intercourse or between periods.*
- Heavier periods.*
- Scanty, erratic or absent periods.*
- Painful periods.*
- Painful sexual intercourse.*
- Bleeding more than one year after periods have ceased in the menopause.*
- Unusual change of odour vaginally.
- Vaginal discharge.

BREASTS

- Tingling, fullness, pain or discomfort.*
- Lumps in the breast or under the armpits.*
- Nipple discharge.*
- Altered breast appearance including dimpled skin or puckered nipples.*

SKIN

● Moles, changing shape, texture, bleeding or discharging, becoming itchy or inflamed.*
● Sudden changes of colour in the skin not due to exposure to weather.*

BOWELS

● Any upset in the bowel routine or the smell of bowel movements.*
● Blood or mucus in the bowel motion.*

BLADDER

● Blood in the urine.*
● Incontinence.*
● Pain on urination.*
● Smelly urine.

PART TWO:

LIFE SPAN

———

Menstruation
Natural contraception
Getting pregnant and pregnancy
Menopause and beyond

CHAPTER 6

MENSTRUATION

——

I've noticed that many women regard their bleeding angrily, distastefully or evasively. You only have to look at the language surrounding menstruation to appreciate this; 'the curse', or more anonymously 'it', 'the time of the month', 'red sails in the sunset', 'coming on', or, as we used to call it at my school 'aunty'. Yet we should be rejoicing when we cross the threshold from childhood into young womanhood. Our menarches (first menstruation) have been happening earlier and earlier. The average age for the first period 150 years ago was seventeen. Now it is thirteen. This is mostly the result of a better diet and healthier living but it is also partly the result of our escalating ingestion of hormones hidden in various foods.

• PUBERTY •

A girl approaching puberty should drink a cup of red raspberry tea in the morning and a cup of blessed thistle tea in the evening, both of which will supply the oestrogen her body will need. The early menstrual cycles usually don't cause the pain and mood changes that later periods can often bring and this may be because a young woman's body is still growing and maturing under the influence of other hormones besides oestrogen. For two or three years after the menarche a girl's body will continue to fill out into adult proportions. By the time she reaches fifteen her face will have lost the round cherubic appearance of a young girl and it will now be restructured by bone and cartilage growth.

• THE MENSTRUAL CYCLE •

Eventually periods settle down into some type of pattern, although there are women who have an irregular period most of their reproductive lives and that is normal for them. Irregular periods, provided you have no other symptoms, rarely indicate that anything is wrong. The odd early, delayed or missed period is nothing to worry about. The rhythm of a woman's menstrual cycle is finely balanced and the slightest thing can throw it out of kilter; stress is a common culprit, as are emotional disturbances such as anxiety and depression. But pregnancy is the commonest cause of missed periods so, when in doubt, have a pregnancy test. The time to seek professional help actively is when you detect a permanent change in your menstrual pattern. If you start to bleed between periods or unpredictably, especially heavily or painfully, or if your periods dry up altogether and you are not in the menopause, seek guidance.

Normally you will lose only about four tablespoonfuls of blood (2 fl oz or 60 ml) over four or five days. The remaining three to four fluid ounces (90 to 120 ml) is made up of water, mucus and other fluids married with fragments of decomposing tissue from the interior of the uterus and several million epithelia cells that flake off the lining of the vagina.

ANAEMIA AND MENSTRUATION

You will need a little extra iron during menstruation as at this time you lose fifteen to thirty mg. Nine out of ten women who have periods are deficient in iron. My favourite iron-rich herbs are raspberry leaves and yellow dock. Drink an infusion of raspberry leaves three times a day. I normally administer yellow dock a tincture; forty drops in the morning and evening. Because tannin will inhibit absorption of yellow dock all tea and coffee should be cut out of the diet while taking this tincture, which is more effective in a little water on an empty stomach. Foods high in iron include anything red, purple or dark green, especially beetroot. One of my favourite juice mixtures is two-thirds freshly pressed carrot and one-third beetroot with a generous plug of raw ginger about the size of half a thumb.

CALCIUM AND MENSTRUATION

The need for calcium increases seven-fold in the week before a period begins. The most easily ingested source of calcium is carrot juice. Drink a glass morning and evening during the course of this week. Other sources of calcium include sprouted wheat, oats, walnuts, hazelnuts, almonds, cabbage, spinach, potatoes, onions and turnips.

Magnesium acts synergistically with calcium and is richly present in many of the same foods as well as beets, dates and sweetcorn.

PAIN AND MENSTRUATION (DYSMENORRHOEA)

It is interesting to note that in more primitive cultures in Central America, China and India, women do not experience any pain with menstruation. The reason why so many women experience menstrual pain in the West is still a much debated subject.

Only twenty per cent of menstrual pain can be accounted for by endometriosis, a retroverted uterus, or some kind of infection. In the remaining eighty per cent it is possible that a uterine contraction feels painful because of pelvic congestion, constipation, spinal lesions which have a specific action on the pelvic organs, weak abdominal tone leading to dropped abdominal and pelvic contents and resulting in congestion and poor circulation or stress. It is not uncommon, for example, for periods to cease altogether following a severe psychological or physical trauma, such as rape. Women who are fearful of getting pregnant are also capable of creating menstrual disorders.

Pain relief

Happily we don't have to know the cause, in this instance, in order to alleviate it. In some women a hot bath and a little alcohol helps, or simply curling up with a hot water bottle. In others ice-packs applied to the abdomen and hot packs supplied to the legs and feet are very helpful to draw blood away from the congested area. I generally assume that if women have menstrual problems their gynaecological organs are not in good condition so I will immediately put them on the formulation on p.114 which is specifically designed to relieve painful menstruation, cramping and irregularities by rebuilding the malfunctioning reproductive system. I also offer simple herbal teas including chamomile, catnip, peppermint, cramp bark or red raspberry. These can be taken in any quantity and are more effective sipped as hot as possible. Also get an osteopath to check your spine, as misalignment of the spiral vertebra can cause womb problems.

Alternate hot and cold sitz baths are an unbeatable way of removing pelvic congestion and restoring ovarian, fallopian and uterine health. These should be taken morning and evening.

Pain immediately before menstruation sometimes suggests that the position of the womb is abnormal. This can sometimes be seen in women who are very thin where the internal fat and ligament upon which the uterus is suspended has lost its tone. A uterus which is tipped towards the spine is called 'retroverted'. One which tips towards the pelvic bone is called 'antiverted'. If it bends over itself it is called 'retroflexed'. There seems to be some sort of gynaecological obsession with uterine positioning, but a tipped uterus is not a condition a woman need worry about. Most women's uteri point in different directions at differing periods of their lives but there are very few women who have a uterus tipped to such an extreme degree that it causes pain or makes any difference in their ability to become pregnant.

However, if the uterus is truly out of position, slant board exercises will help (see Appendix 3), as will the simple acts of walking, swimming or yoga. The Kegal exercises on p.92 are also invaluable. Sometimes severe Candida can contribute to menstrual pain, so it is worth having this checked out.

EXERCISES FOR MENSTRUAL PAIN

I know it is very tempting to creep into bed hugging a hot water bottle and feeling sorry for yourself, but try and do at least one of the following exercises, if not the whole series.

1. Lie on your back at right angles to the wall, with your buttocks as near to the wall as possible. Prop your feet up against the wall, making sure that the soles are flat and the knees are a little bent. Maintain this position for five minutes.
2. While lying down and having moved away from the wall, bring one leg

up as close to your chin as you can get it, leaving the other flat on the floor. Hold the lifted leg up with your arms and maintain that position for two minutes then repeat it using the other leg.

3. Get up so that you are resting on your knees and elbows and stretching your head and arms out so that your elbows are on the ground in front of you and your head is between your arms. Hold this position for two minutes. This is particularly helpful for those who have pain immediately after intercourse and just before a period is due.

4. The cobra. This is a yogic position in which you begin by lying face down flat on the floor and then gradually raise your head and chest without using your arms. Then, now using the arms, continue to raise your chest until your back is arched and your head is bent back as far as possible with your eyes cast back looking above you. Inhale as you raise your body and exhale when you lower your trunk to the floor. Do this slowly. Relax and repeat (once only).

5. The bow. This is a yogic posture in which you lie face down, bend your knees, grab your ankles with your hands and then release and relax. Inhale as you begin and exhale after release. If you are flexible you can also rock back and forth on your stomach in the bow position while holding your breath.

6. Acupressure points will also help to relieve lower back pain. Lie face-down on a hard surface and have a companion press with the flat of the thumb along the sides of each vertebrae from the tail of the spine up to the waist. Hold each pressure point to the count of ten and then slowly release.

7. One of the most pleasant methods of relieving cramps is to have an orgasm, but masturbating in order to achieve this while you are in great pain may, understandably, be out of the question.

• THE COLOUR OF BLOOD •

If menstrual blood is bright red it is indicative of poor absorption and digestion of sugar and carbohydrates. If it is dark red, stringy or smelly it shows that the body is overburdened with putrefying protein and you should cut right back on all meats, eggs and dairy products. The ideal colour of healthy menstrual blood is reddish brown and it should flow easily and freely.

• EXCESSIVELY HEAVY PERIODS (MENORRHAGIA) •

If you suffer from very heavy periods it is worth going for a thorough check-up to identify the cause. Heavy bleeding may be a symptom of fibroids, endometriosis or pelvic infection. There may also be emotional causes for heavy bleeding, notably depression. Women who have been sterilised sometimes complain of menorrhagia.

REFLEXOLOGY

Reflexology can often be very successful in treating heavy periods and you can do this yourself.

- Sit comfortably on a couch and put your foot in your lap so that you can easily reach the sides. The reflexology pressure points for the genitals and female organs are around the ankle.
- Press on the inside of your foot with the flat of your thumb on a spot about half way between your ankle-bone and the bottom of your heel. This is the uterine point.
- Press on a similar spot on the outside of your foot, the ovaries.
- Squeeze and pinch either side of your Achilles tendon about three inches (7.5 cm) up from your heel. This will also affect the uterus. If it feels tender or hurts go gently but don't stop.
- Work on these points throughout the month but not during the actual flow as this will make it even heavier.

FASTING

Fasting on the first day of a heavy flow, or the day before the period begins, certainly helps. Take ten drops hourly of tormentavena (see Resources Directory). Alternatively, take between twenty and fifty drops twice a day of horsetail tincture or Bioforce's Tormentavena throughout the entire month. Continue, if necessary, for several months until the bleeding is lighter. Do the liver flush on p.63. The liver plays a great part in hormonal regulation. Make sure that you have an abundance of iron and calcium in your diet.

• LACK OF PERIODS (AMENORRHOEA) •

While it is common for the initial periods following the menarche to be irregular, the absence of periods is usually the result of stress, an extreme diet, including fruitarianism, or too much exercise. If you are very thin, try to put on weight.

Between forty and sixty drops of chaste tree tincture morning and evening on an empty stomach can be helpful to bring on periods, as can the same dosage of Chinese angelica. Other herbs which may help include blue cohosh, black cohosh, false unicorn, licorice or holy thistle. All of these may be taken as teas.

• BLEEDING BETWEEN PERIODS AND AFTER INTERCOURSE •

Seek medical advice.

• WATER RETENTION •

Water retention, or Oedema (see p.129), is common as part of premenstrual tension just before a period but can happen at any time due to the levels of certain hormones in the body. Common symptoms are breast tenderness, a swollen abdomen, headaches, constipation, irritability, and swelling in the ankles, feet, hands or face. If you are not sure if you have oedema, press your thumb against your shin-bone for twenty seconds. If after removing it you notice a white indented area which fails to fill up within five seconds and return to your normal colouring, you have water retention. If this is the case it may take up to two minutes for the white area and the indentation to normalise.

One of the safest and most delicious teas you can take to help yourself is roasted dandelion root which can be prepared as a coffee. Delicious if made as a decoction and drunk black with a touch of honey, if desired, it is rich in potassium so unlike medical diuretics it does not leach potassium from the system.

Cut out all forms of salt from the diet including hidden salt in processed food (see page 13). Those foods that are rich in vitamin C increase urine flow which helps to alleviate symptoms. The kidney tea on page 65 is also an excellent and safe diuretic.

• LEG CRAMPS •

If you suffer with leg cramps, ensure you are taking plenty of calcium in its natural form to relieve the pain and nourish the muscles. Also take ten drops three times a day of ginkgo biloba and ten drops three times a day of Bioforce's Petesan (see Resources Directory) together with foods richly abundant in vitamin E (which include wholegrains and the oils extracted from them, as well as nuts and seeds). Cold water walking in the bath often helps (simply walking in a bath which is full of cold water, reaching almost up to the knee) as do the methods on p.185.

• HYPOGLYCAEMIA •

Hypoglycaemia, low blood sugar level, is extremely wide spread and often manifests in menstruating women. I would estimate that some sixty per cent of my patients suffer from it to some degree or another. Unhappily it is often undiagnosed and its multitude of symptoms are labelled merely emotional or psychological.

BLOOD GLUCOSE LEVELS

Usually blood glucose levels are stabilised within a narrow band of variation by different hormones which react rapidly to the slightest changes. Insulin from the pancreas is released when glucose enters the blood from digested foods, so the blood glucose level remains normal. The sugar is then stored in the liver and muscles as glycogen, or is converted to fat for later use. Cortisol and growth hormone counterbalance such insulin action. If any of these hormones are secreted too quickly or too slowly the blood glucose level (BGL) becomes imbalanced. The most commonly involved glands and organs in this hypoglycaemic roller coaster are the adrenals, pancreas and liver. Hypoglycaemia is sometimes caused by a diet too rich in refined carbohydrates and adrenalin-producing caffeine, as well as stress. Caffeine stimulates the adrenal glands which try to mobilise the body's energy reserves in the liver and muscles so removing its fail-safe mechanism for keeping the BGL in balance.

DIAGNOSIS

Hypoglycaemia can be accurately diagnosed using a five-hour blood glucose tolerance test. Symptoms include irritability, fatigue, depression, an insatiable craving for sweets or carbohydrates, inability to concentrate, sweating, shaking, palpitations, tingling of the skin, lips or scalp, dizziness, trembling, fainting, blurred vision, nausea, rapid swoops and dips in energy particularly in the middle of the morning and mid-to late-afternoon, anxiety, indecisiveness and crying. Symptoms are usually improved by eating.

DIET

The best diet to follow if you suffer with hypoglycaemia is a high fibre carbohydrate diet with adequate sources of non-animal protein in it. Meals should be small and spread out over the course of a day. Food should be unrefined and slow to digest.

Fruit

Dried fruit, fresh fruit, freshly pressed fruit juices and vegetable juices are all rapidly absorbed and therefore should be consumed moderately. It is advisable to dilute fruit and vegetable juices half and half with purified water. When eating fruit, it should be taken with a handful of nuts or soya yogurt. Fruit juice can be further fortified by superfoods high in protein including spirulina, chlorella and nutritional yeast.

Nutritional yeast

Nutritional yeast is particularly abundant in glucose tolerance factor (foods which help to stabilise glucose levels in the system) of which chromium is king. Take a desert spoon of this three times a day. It is essential for carbohydrate metabolism and proper insulin function.

Fibre

Fibre will help the regular absorption of carbohydrate from the intestine. Foods which are particularly useful include whole grains, especially presoaked and low-heated oats, nuts, nut butters and nut milks, avocado, nutritional yeast and Jerusalem artichokes. It is important to avoid sugar in all its forms absolutely. Once the blood sugar levels have been thoroughly stabilised you can introduce a teaspoonful or two of maple syrup daily. Anything refined should be avoided as should alcohol, coffee and cigarettes. Use whatever methods work for you for stress control and eat only when relaxed.

Many women with menstrual problems find following a hypoglycaemic diet extremely helpful.

• PREMENSTRUAL SYNDROME (PMS) •

The highest number of violent crimes committed by women take place in the four to seven days prior to menstruation. These days are also the peak times for women being admitted to both prison and psychiatric institutions. Shop lifting is thirty times more common at this time and there is also a bigger percentage of female accidents and suicide attempts than at other times. Brain waves in the premenstrual period are increased in frequency and amplitude compared to those of mid-cycle. All of which is proof, if proof were needed, of the physiological and psychological alteration that takes place before a period.

PHYSICAL AND EMOTIONAL SYMPTOMS

Many of the physical changes manifested during PMS are the results of a shift in fluid balance in response to progesterone which is produced in large quantities after ovulation. Physical changes may include swelling of the breasts, feet and hands, haemorrhoids, abdominal bloating, weight gain, migraines, backache, cramping, painful joints, marred skin and lank hair, asthma, hay fever, hoarseness, nausea and red eyes. Emotional problems may include food or alcohol cravings, depression, loss of concentration, fatigue and irritability.

DIET

A hypoglycaemic diet is ideal for PMS sufferers. The craving for refined carbohydrates including sugar increases tremendously with PMS. It seems it is not the hypoglycaemic state itself that causes PMS because symptoms of hypoglycaemia disappear soon after food is eaten; in any case, hypoglycaemia never lasts for days on end. What hypoglycaemia does is to overburden the adrenal glands as they struggle to stabilise drastically fluctuating blood sugar levels. Distressed adrenal glands need an abundance of vitamin B-complex and vitamin C.

These vitamins are essential for carbohydrate metabolism and are often missing in a typical Western diet of highly refined carbohydrate – a diet which produces hypoglycaemia in the first place. So women with refined carbohydrate cravings get stuck in a vicious cycle alternately producing hypoglycaemia and adrenal exhaustion. This is why B-complex and B6 have been so successful in treating certain cases of PMS.

Many PMS sufferers eat four-and-a-half times more dairy products than women who escape this syndrome. Saturated animal fat inhibits the formation of PGE1, which is an anti-inflammatory prostaglandin deficient in PMS sufferers. Evening primrose oil, blackcurrant or borage oil all enhance the production of PGE1. They are all oils rich in gammalinoleic acid (GLA) and must be taken at a minimum dose of 1,500 mg every day of the month. Vitamin E is also useful as an inhibitor against the formation of a PGE antagonist derived from meat.

Other ways to help

Osteopathic adjustment may be necessary to relieve bloating, and exercise certainly helps.

DIFFERENT TYPES OF PMS

There is not one, but four different types of PMS. Women with PMS-A have abnormal hormone levels too high in oestrogen and low in progesterone, and suffer from anxiety, irritability and nervous tension as a result. PMS-H women have water retention problems with subsequent bloating and breast pain. PMS-C women crave refined carbohydrates and feel weak and headachey. PMS-D women can get profoundly depressed, forgetful and confused, for them progesterone levels are too high and oestrogen is too low. Women with PMS-A tend to eat large amounts of dairy produce, while those with PMS-H eat too much refined carbohydrate and those with PMS-C too much animal fat. PMS-D women are especially vulnerable to the affects of environmental lead. All PMS sufferers are deficient in B-complex vitamins and magnesium, both of which are closely involved with the mood-altering chemicals in the brain. A magnesium deficiency is exacerbated by a diet high in dairy products which also allows more lead to get into the body.

I have found that severe Candida can exacerbate PMS so it is worth investigating.

Apart from following all the advice on a hypoglycaemic diet on pages 111–12 take the following precrash tonic in the ten days leading up to your period.

Precrash Tonic

Equal parts:
chaste tree
wild yam
sarsaparilla
dandelion
valerian
uva ursi

corn silk
false unicorn
squawvine
blue cohosh
cramp bark
sage
ginger
blessed thistle

Make as a tincture and take fifteen drops three times a day in a little water. Once the period starts switch to the female corrective formulation below. Or use Boiron's or Boericke & Tafel's PMS formulas.

I found this an extremely successful formulation if followed faithfully over a period of some months, together with the preceding advice.

Female Corrective

This combination of herbs helps to rebuild a malfunctioning reproductive system and is an excellent general tonic. It nourishes the malfunctioning organs.

Equal parts of: *false unicorn*
goldenseal root   *ginger*
blessed thistle   *red raspberry*
cayenne   *squawvine*
cramp bark   *uva ursi*

Decoct and drink three cups a day.

CHAPTER 7:

NATURAL CONTRACEPTION

There is a 3,500-year-old reference that was discovered on an Egyptian papyrus to a method of contraception which demanded that a mixture of sodium carbonate, honey and crocodile dung be mixed as a paste and inserted into the vagina before intercourse. This mixture inhibits sperm mobility but the Egyptians could not know that because sperm hadn't yet been discovered!

• THE DIAPHRAGM •

Casanova is credited with developing the first cervical cap or diaphragm. Apparently, he grabbed the first thing that came to hand, a lemon, sliced it in half, hollowed it out and placed it over his partner's cervix! He then graduated to the use of gold balls to seal off the uterine opening (because presumably lemons weren't always handy) and this remained the fashionable method of choice until late 1800 when a German physician developed the first rubber dome diaphragm. The diaphragm remains as reliable today as ever it was, providing it is properly used. As well as protecting from pregnancy, it has the added advantage of protecting the cervix from developing cancer and helps to reduce the risk of pelvic infection and HIV (the AIDS virus is thought to be destroyed by spermicides). Nor does it have any of the serious side-effects of the pill or IUD. However, cystitis is more common with diaphragm users and I have known some women to develop an allergy to the spermicide. It also makes spontaneous sex virtually impossible.

• THE CONDOM •

The Romans used animal bladders as condoms to prevent the transfer of sexually transmitted disease; by the eighteenth century sheep's bowel was used instead. Once rubber technology developed sufficiently, the condom made a dramatic contribution to contraception and now between thirty and forty million couples use it. Properly used, the failure rate is only two or three per cent and the advantages are that condom protects the cervix from cervical cancer and cervical infection, reducing the chance of contracting sexually transmitted diseases, including HIV. It reduces the man's stimulation, so prolonging intercourse which can contribute towards a woman achieving orgasm. Disadvantages include a slight lack of spontaneity; some people complain about them smelling odd; and certainly they are very hard to flush away down the toilet. Wrapping them up and incinerating them after use would be kinder to the environment.

• THE INTRA-UTERINE DEVICE (IUD) •

By the 1900s intra-uterine devices were being tried, made out of glass, wood, ivory, silver and gold. However, they had to be abandoned because they caused infection or bleeding. Newer models made out of plastic shaped into loops, coils or T-shapes seemed to work better although no one could understand why. Some feel that an IUD acts as an irritant in the uterus and the uterine lining becomes altered in response to the irritation so that implantation cannot take place, while others feel that white blood cells speed to the irritated lining just as they would to an infection and, in their attempt to destroy the IUD, they also destroy the embryo if one should appear.

DISADVANTAGES

The disadvantages are heavier, more painful periods for ten per cent of the women fitted with IUDs, heavier discharge or even persistent thrush. The IUD does not protect against sexually transmitted diseases including HIV, and there is a higher risk of ectopic pregnancy.

My own feeling is that IUDs are almost as harmful as the pill. Not only is their failure rate higher than that of the pill (4.1 per cent against 3 per cent) but the side-effects, for those unfortunate enough to experience them, can be horrific.

FINAL THOUGHTS

Of these two approaches, the diaphragm versus the sheath (or any method similar to the diaphragm, including the customised cap and the sponge), I would favour the sheath. In my own practice I have found a large number of women react to the toxic and irritating affects of spermicidal chemicals which can easily enter the blood-stream and so distress the whole body. Internally or externally, chemicals should always be approached with caution.

• THE PILL •

I am also in total support of Dr Ellen Grant who, in her book *The Bitter Pill*, damns the contraceptive pill beyond redemption. She links it to cancer, thrombosis, migraine, food allergies and hyperactive and dyslexic children. In fact evidence against the Pill from very many reliable and respectable quarters is now so huge that I encourage my patients to stay clear of it as far as they possibly can (see Appendix 1, page 211). Paavo Airola, in his excellent *Every Woman's Book*, presents an enormous list of the less serious side-effects of oral contraceptives and these include:

- increased susceptibility to vaginal and bladder infections;
- lowered resistance to all infections;
- cramps;
- dry, blotchy skin;
- mouth ulcers;
- dry, falling hair and baldness;
- premature wrinkling;
- acne;
- sleep disturbances;
- inability to concentrate;
- migraine headaches;
- depression, moodiness, irritability;
- darkening of the skin, of the upper lip, and lower eye lids;
- sore breasts;
- nausea;
- weight gain and body distortion due to disproportional distribution of fat;
- chronic fatigue;
- increase in dental cavities;
- swollen and bleeding gums;
- greatly increased or decreased sex drive;
- visual disturbances;
- amenorrhoea;
- blood sugar disturbances which complicate diabetes or hypoglycaemia.

The more serious complaints caused by oral contraceptives he lists as:

- eczema;
- gall-bladder problems;
- hyperlipemia (excess fat in the blood);
- intolerance to carbohydrates leading to 'steroid diabetes', which can lead to clinical diabetes;
- strokes;
- seven to ten times greater risk of death due to blood clots;
- jaundice, liver damage and liver tumours;
- epilepsy;
- high blood pressure;
- kidney failure;
- oedema;
- permanent infertility;
- varicose veins;
- thrombophlebitis and pulmonary embolism;
- heart attacks;
- cancer of the breast, uterus, liver and pituitary gland.

As far as I am concerned there is no contest. Besides which, the Pill has been well proven to deplete the body nutritionally.

• STERILISATION •

This is, of course, almost one hundred per cent foolproof but there is some evidence that the operation can interfere with the blood supply to the ovaries and so with the production of hormones lead to excessively heavy periods. So common are the complaints after sterilisation, some gynaecologists have begun to use the term 'post-tubal ligation syndrome' to describe pain with intercourse, pelvic pain or a feeling of pressure, cramping, heavy periods and bleeding between periods.

Some theories suggest that the cutting off of the blood supply to the ovaries can cause endometriosis, and the extra pressure of the backed-up blood can alter a woman's hormonal balance. These problems are believed to get worse with time. A recent study suggested that women who had been sterilised are three times more likely to have a hysterectomy than women who haven't.

• NATURAL FAMILY PLANNING •

I feel that the inconvenience presented by barrier contraception, including the condom or the diaphragm or even natural family planning, is a small price to pay compared to the pain and difficulties associated with everything else that medicine has so far come up with, including IUDs, the Pill and sterilisation.

Twenty years ago the whole idea of natural family planning was simply a joke. Proponents of natural family planning in the sophisticated and accurate way in which it is now taught say that this method is extremely effective if couples simply follow the rules faithfully. However, if you are to use the method confidently and successfully you do need special instruction from a trained teacher, particularly if your periods are irregular, if you are breast feeding or nearing the menopause.

Proponents claim a ninety-nine per cent success rate, however, some small things can upset the reading of the cervical mucus. These include: an infection which can increase the temperature and so mask a raise that signals ovulation; alcohol, which can do the same thing; vaginal infections and semen left in the vagina from previous intercourse which can make mucus signs more difficult to interpret; or stress.

• VITAMIN C •

In Russia, Vitamin C has been found to be ninety-six per cent effective as a contraceptive. The tablet is inserted into the vagina ten minutes before intercourse and its contraceptive effects are believed to last for half an hour. American research suggests that this can only be used safely coupled with cyclic methods of natural birth control.

• HERBS •

The Indian tribes in Nevada have been drinking a tea made from the roots and seeds of Lithosperma for centuries to prevent contraception. It inhibits the action of gonadotrophin on the ovaries. Cherokee women use Cicuta maculata and, if taken four days in succession, it results in permanent sterility. Moroccan women are reported to eat raw castor beans, one for each year they wish to remain infertile, with success, and castor beans are used for the same purpose in other parts of Africa and in India.

Other herbs which are believed to act as contraceptives include milkweed, Indian turnip, ragleaf, bahia, cramp bark, dogbane, wild yam, stoneseed and false hellebore. On reflection I wouldn't recommend any of these. Just because it is natural it doesn't mean it is not toxic. These herbs seem to work by poisoning the whole body, so making it unfit for reproduction. Sterility is nature's way of preserving the quality and life of the species. Some of these herbs, while not necessarily toxic in themselves, are taken in amounts so great they alter and interfere with the body's basic biochemical and hormonal cycles and, in my opinion, they are no better than the Pill.

Overall, I would recommend using barrier methods. However, if natural family planning is expertly taught and properly followed, this is the method I favour most of all.

CHAPTER 8:

GETTING PREGNANT AND PREGNANCY

———

The Bible tells us that the sins of the fathers are visited on the children, which might be interpreted as saying that we pass on our genetic blueprints to our children. Sadly, they tend to get scruffier as they go down the line. If your children suffer allergies, asthma or hay fever, if they have to wear glasses or have a mouth full of fillings inspite of a reasonable diet, the chances are that you, your parents and even your grandparents were lacking in adequate nutrition and this problem will have been exacerbated generation after generation. The good news is you can change the pattern by looking after your own state of health **well before** you conceive. I ask those I work with to allow a minimum of six months to prepare for a really healthy conception. During this time an unhealthy lifestyle which may involve a rubbishy diet, smoking, heavy drinking, drugs, weight problems or lack of exercise, as well as high stress levels, can be altered.

It is advisable not to become pregnant until you have been off the Pill for three to six months. Cleansing the traces of the Pill out of your system is vital. Among its many other problems the Pill lowers levels of folic acid. Inadequate folic acid in the system has been linked to spina bifida. Women who stop taking the Pill and who conceive within six months of this time have a reduced blood cell count and plasma foliate levels in the first three months of their pregnancy. Some cellular abnormalities of the cervix are also linked to impaired status of folic acid. So a woman coming off the Pill needs a truly excellent diet to help her get her system back to normal. Post Pill amenorrhoea is common (for help see p.109).

• PRE-CONCEPTION CLEANSING •

Once you have decided to try to conceive, short, regular fasts of either fruit or vegetable juices are recommended, coupled with a diet which is as near to vegan as you can get it. If you are eating flesh products ensure that they are organic.

Men should give up smoking and drinking in order to improve both the quality and quantity of sperm. Some authorities recommend adhering to the marital requirements in the Old Testament, which prohibits sexual intercourse during menstruation and for a week afterwards. It is argued that this regime encourages intercourse at times of highest female fertility and it builds up a man's sperm count so that there is a better chance of fertilisation. It also increases the health of the prospective mother by giving her gynaecological organs a chance to regulate themselves during her cycle. If the father eats a diet high in Vitamin E on a regular basis for many months before conception this might have beneficial effects on the development of the foetus's brain.

• HERBS •

Any of the following herbs, taken as an infusion or decoction, will help to tone and balance the body gynaecologically:

- red raspberry leaf (infusion)
- squawvine (decoction)
- blessed thistle (decoction);
- false unicorn (decoction – an excellent tonic for both male and female reproductive organs);
- true unicorn root (decoction).

MALE ENERGY TONIC

Just as its name suggests, this tonic will increase a man's potency.

Two parts: *damiana*
Siberian ginseng root   *saw palmetto berry*
Korean ginseng root   *oat seed*
One part: *cardamom seed*
sarsaparilla

This can be made as a tincture, in which case the dose is fifteen drops three times a day, or brewed as a decoction, in which case the dosage is a cup with every meal.

To ensure prostate health make sure the bowel and lymphatic systems are clean – consider asking an iridologist for advice. In addition take Bioforce's Prostasan in tincture form, fifteen drops three times a day before meals.

Pumpkin seeds are rich in a male androgen hormone which will help to cleanse the prostate gland. Eat a couple of ounces every day.

• THE IMPORTANCE OF EXERCISE •

WOMEN

Women should concentrate on exercises that strengthen the muscles of the pelvic floor (see p.92) as well as some form of enjoyable aerobic exercise. Do not over-exercise as this may result in amenorrhoea (see p.109).

MEN

Men should take regular exercise too. Remember everybody's most important nutritional requirement is oxygen. Sedentary lifestyles lead to chronic oxygen starvation. Exercise should be taken outdoors in the purest, cleanest air you can find, a tall order nowadays, I know. Forty minutes of vigorous exercise three times a week is adequate.

• SUBFERTILITY •

This seems to be on the rise and may be tied to increasing pollution, both internal and external. A very common cause of female infertility is blocked or partly blocked fallopian tubes, which can be the result of previously undetected pelvic infections.

About twenty-five per cent of all couples conceive the first month they try; fifty per cent will have succeeded within six months, and eighty-five per cent within a year. Of the remaining fifteen per cent, one-quarter will conceive in the following year. Nevertheless investigation after one year is probably wise. Amongst couples who do have problems conceiving, in about forty per cent of cases the problem is due to the male partner and usually the trouble is one of low sperm count.

SPERM

Impaired sperm production in a man can be the result of heavy metal poisoning, radiation exposure or prolonged drug use as well as an undetected infection leading to atrophy of the testicles, or a trauma or blow to the testicles. Obstruction of the seminal tract itself may be congenital or due to inflammation of the prostate, inflammation of the testicles or any other local inflammatory process.

With repeated ejaculations the number of sperm in the ejaculate decline, so if your partner has ejaculated several times over the preceding few days, conception is less likely to occur on the day you ovulate because his semen will contain insufficient sperm. For this reason it is probably best to abstain from intercourse for two to three days before ovulation is expected to occur. If a woman stands up and walks around immediately after making love most of the seminal fluid will leak out of her vagina. To give as many sperm as possible a chance of reaching the fallopian tubes where the egg cell will be, it is a sensible idea to lie quietly on the bed for at least twenty minutes after making love with the buttocks raised slightly on a pillow and the knees bent upwards.

TREATMENT

I have had an enormous amount of success in this area using a holistic approach. From my own experience I have found too many subfertile couples think only of their reproductive organs when the problem is likely to be far more wide ranging. Treatment normally includes systemic detoxification. I will often suggest short vegetable juice fasts of five consecutive days every fortnight coupled with a vegan diet, which includes plenty of raw and sprouted food. In cases where nothing can be found to prevent conception in either partner, I will often use the following programme, or a modification of this programme.

The Intensive Detox Programme

The diet must be one hundred per cent vegan and should include all vegetables, fruits, raw nuts and seeds, presoaked and low heated grains and sprouted grains and beans. Eat fresh organic produce that is grown locally and in season if at all possible. Use only filtered water, herbal teas and freshly pressed fruit and vegetable juices. Organic juices which are bottled are also permissible. Take no cooked foods at all (bread, baked potatoes, tofu, etc). Absolutely no alcohol, coffee, tea, sugar or salt.

I add to this the female corrective (p.114) and use specific superfoods depending on the outcome of a vega or iridology test. I have found hydrotherapy particularly useful. Hot and cold sitz baths of plain water, morning and evening for both men and women remove internal inflammation and ingestion. At the very least patients are asked to take alternative hot and cold sitz baths morning and evening.

TEMPERATURE CHARTS

If you have been trying unsuccessfully to conceive for more than six months and you are under thirty, check that you are not consistently making love on infertile days of the month by using a temperature chart and detecting the change in your cervical mucus (a kit can be purchased from the Wholistic Research Company whose address is listed in the Resources Directory). A woman's natural fertility tends to decline after the age of thirty but if you have had a child or a previous pregnancy and are unable to conceive you both need to seek a complete diagnostic evaluation.

• PREGNANCY •

Pregnancy and birth are normal physiological processes. Pregnancy is not an illness. Birth does not usually require instruments, tubing, chemicals, drugs, machines or doctors. The prevailing attitude in the Western world that doctors deliver babies, rather than the belief that women give birth, continues to encourage a high rate of medical intervention (including episiotomies, forceps or vacuum extracted deliveries and caesareans). True reasons for intervention are very few indeed and should be reserved for the rare occasions when otherwise the safety of the mother or baby would be put at risk.

This may sound radical, even unpalatable to some, but I believe that hospitals are not the safest place to give birth. In Holland, where pregnant women may choose whether a doctor or a midwife attends them and where, it has emerged that the safest option of all is a home birth with a midwife. This is true even for first-time mothers.

Prenatal care focuses on screening for problems to such a degree that the ability to diagnose defects has far outpaced the possibility of curing them or even accurately describing how they will affect the baby. Advances in technology can themselves be dangerous and carry with them anguish, uncertainty, inaccuracy and some hard choices. The poor foetus, let us not forget what pregnancy is all about, becomes an unborn patient.

DIET DURING PREGNANCY

Excellent nutrition helps every single aspect of conception, pregnancy and birth. It lowers the risk of everything from low birth weight, prematurity and eclampsia to caesarean sections and has been proved to result in fewer stillbirths, better brain development, fewer learning disabilities and healthier babies. During the Second World War, British women were given priority in the food rationing restrictions and even under these adverse conditions the stillbirth rate fell from thirty-eight per 1,000 live births to twenty-eight, a drop of almost twenty-five per cent.

I do not recommend vitamin and mineral supplements made synthetically for the reasons outlined on pages 24–5.

Folic Acid

Since 1991 women planning to become pregnant have been advised by the British Government to take supplements of folic acid, however, it is richly present in dark green leafy vegetables, organic nutritional yeast and dates. Ample helpings of broccoli or any other dark green leafy vegetable such as spinach, as well as one or two dried dates every day, will ensure the recommended 400 mg intake daily throughout pregnancy.

B6

Excessive vitamin B6 can be toxic to mother and baby but it is present in its natural form in green vegetables, grains, pulses and nutritional yeast. It is essential for vital energy-producing reactions as well as healthy nerves and mucous membranes. Taken in its natural form you cannot overdose on it because the body will simply dispose of what it doesn't need.

Vitamin D

Excessive synthetic vitamin D can be toxic to mother and baby. Vitamin D enriched soya milks are available, but fifteen minutes' walk outside exposing your face and arms daily is all that is required to meet pregnancy needs. Vitamin D is stored in the liver so a summer of gentle sunshine and moderate exposure to it should create all the body's supplies, certainly enough to carry it throughout the winter.

Iron

The need for iron during pregnancy escalates greatly simply because mother and baby are busy creating large quantities of new blood. A non-pregnant woman requires only 18 mg of iron a day but a pregnant woman can need as much as 42 mg per day. There is large variation because of huge differences among women in the efficiency of their absorption of iron from the intestine into the bloodstream. On average women absorb ten per cent of the iron they consume.

Dairy products actually inhibit the absorption of iron. The use of dairy products undermines the use of greens and other iron-rich plant foods.

Women who are good absorbers of iron should get sufficient supply from green leafy vegetables, raisins, whole grains and foods made from whole grains as well as nuts, seeds, pulses, molasses and dried fruit.

Vitamin C greatly increases the absorption of iron from food into the bloodstream, so green leafy vegetables which are abundant in both iron and vitamin C are especially valuable during pregnancy. For example 60 mg of vitamin C increases the absorption of iron in corn by five times. Therefore, vitamin C-containing foods, such as broccoli, brussels sprouts, potatoes, sweet potatoes, peppers, tomatoes and cabbage, are especially good to combine with iron-rich foods.

Excessive iron taken in its synthetic form can cause stomach irritation and can be toxic to both the mother and the baby.

Zinc

This is essential for the baby as well as the health of the pregnant mother and is richly present in whole grains, green leafy vegetables, mushrooms, nuts, seeds (especially sesame-tahini), pulses, tofu, misi, wheatgerm and nutritional yeast. A zinc-rich diet will help to protect the skin from stretch marks.

Calcium

The body's ability to absorb calcium is directly dependent upon the amount of phosphorus in the diet. The lower the level of phosphorus, the harder it is to absorb calcium. Foods where the phosphorus ratio is low and therefore the calcium is least available are meat and fish. Magnesium is also essential for the proper assimilation of calcium – the ideal ratio is five parts calcium to three parts magnesium. All the plant foods previously mentioned in the sections on zinc and iron have this in perfect ratio.

Pregnant women need 1,000 mg of calcium daily. To ensure adequate daily supplies of calcium in pregnancy it only takes three servings of one of the following: 8 fl oz of carrot juice, 4 oz of broccoli or a level tablespoonful of tahini.

Vitamin B12

This vitamin is necessary for normal blood cell growth and nerve function. It is needed only in tiny amounts; an average of three millionths of a gram every day is sufficient for all adults, whether pregnant or not. The liver is able to store three to five years' supply of vitamin B12 and this acts as a great B12 buffer for the body. Consequently, there is absolutely no need to ingest the vitamin daily.

No animal makes B12. It is made by bacteria that grow in the soil and in fermented foods. There are bacteria within the human body that make vitamin B12, in the mouth, saliva, in the liver's bile, and within the intestinal contents.

B12 is present in virtually all sprouted seeds, particularly alfalfa. It is also found in high levels in many herbs including comfrey, garlic, parsley and chlorella, spirulina and nutritional yeast. If you maintain optimal intestinal health (see p.67–74) the small intestines are capable of manufacturing their own B12. Fermented foods like tempeh, miso and shoyu are also rich in B12.

Iodine

Deficiency of iodine in pregnancy increases the risk of stillbirth. Pregnant women can safely take 3 mg a day, which should ideally be obtained from safe natural sources such as seaweeds.

Vitamin K

If the intestinal bacteria are healthy they generally produce sufficient vitamin K, but because this vitamin is fat-soluble it cannot easily pass through the placenta into the blood of your baby. Newborn babies do not have the intestinal bacteria which manufacture vitamin K. Natural sources of vitamin K include kelp and other seaweeds, alfalfa, all dark green leafy vegetables, black strap molasses, apricots, sunflower seeds and their oil and garlic. Supplementation for the baby is not necessary while breast feeding if the mother's diet is abundant in these foods.

Pregnancy Tea

This consists of equal parts of red raspberry leaves, squawvine, nettles, thyme, alfalfa and red clover. Drink a cup morning and evening throughout the course of your pregnancy. This combination provides nutrients that are necessary for a good strong pregnancy. Raspberry leaves contain fragarine which will help both pregnancy and birth, as well as citrate of iron in a digestible form. Alfalfa is full of minerals and is rich in vitamin K.

• EXERCISE •

Exercise is vital throughout pregnancy. If you suffer from morning sickness it is tempting to do nothing and your exercise programme will often be forgotten for the rest of your pregnancy. However, if you actively participated in some exercise before conception you can usually continue, although you need to use your common sense and take advice if you are worried.

If you begin to feel too heavy to exercise properly, still continue to do what you can. Swimming is one of the best activities for pregnant women; the water buoys the tummy up, the whole body is exercised and it can be continued right up until birth.

It is inspiring to note that during the Second World War women had to take over the job of railway porters from men and those who took the jobs had no problem with birthing. Their less active sisters were not always so lucky.

Yoga is particularly recommended, not simply because it includes several special exercises for the pelvis, but also because it leads to increased poise, self-confidence, better physical co-ordination and a wonderful internal sense of serenity and balance.

• THE IMPORTANCE OF TOUCH •

Touch is becoming increasingly important in our straight-jacketed Western cultures where we seldom get enough of it. It takes twelve hugs a day to optimise your immune system. Societies that give their babies the greatest amount of physical affection and touching have the lowest level of physical abuse. So give and receive plenty of touch including bodywork (any work done on the body, such as Swedish massage, hellework, reflexology or aromatherapy) of your choice.

• HERBS •

Intake of herbs needs to be very strictly controlled in the first three months of pregnancy (but the pregnancy tea I have given you is perfectly safe) and I will never put a pregnant woman through any kind of deep cleansing programme.

The herbs that should not be taken during pregnancy are:

aloe, broom, celery, coltsfoot, cramp bark, false unicorn, heartsease, licorice, nutmeg, pennyroyal, sassafras, shepherd's purse, tansy.

• MEDICINES •

Whilst pregnant do not take any drugs, except under strict medical supervision. Use natural alternatives especially in the first three months, if necessary.

These should be administered externally as hand/foot/sitz and full baths. Drugs can cross the placenta and can damage the foetus.

• SMOKING •

It has now been suggested that foetal heartbeat can accelerate through anxiety, even when the mother is only thinking of having a cigarette. This is not surprising. The reduction of oxygen in the baby's blood supply, the baby's only lifeline, must produce a very unpleasant feeling.

• ALCOHOL •

Alcohol is rapidly absorbed into the bloodstream and can cross the placenta to befuddle the baby and make her less active in the womb than she should be. It is best to avoid alcohol in pregnancy.

• MORNING SICKNESS •

Some herbalists believe that chemical by-products of the hormonal changes in the body can cause morning sickness. Walking daily will help to eliminate these chemicals and of course you need to eat correctly so avoid adding them to your system. Foods to avoid are anything white or refined, especially sugar, as well as high levels of animal protein. Chlorophyll, if necessary injected rectally, will help to prevent chemical build up.

Other herbalists believe that excessive protein requirements of the developing baby can cause morning sickness and, if this is the case, small frequent snacks of protein-rich and easily digestible food are said to help (providing you can keep them down). A wholefood diet which is high in carbohydrate, fresh fruit, lightly steamed and raw vegetables, and protein-rich foods is ideal. Spirulina, chlorella and nutritional yeasts are particularly indicated in pregnancy. Stomach acids can be neutralised by eating a peeled apple. Many women tell me that if they move around slowly they can avert an attack of morning sickness. In extreme cases I have found acupuncture can help.

Ginger tea liberally laced with honey and lemon has been the most effective cure that I have found. The good news is that almost all morning sickness stops by the fourth month of pregnancy.

• CRAMPS DURING PREGNANCY •

Womb cramping or false labour pains may be treated with a chamomile poultice applied to the abdomen or a daily dose of one or two cups of cramp bark decoction sipped hot. Use 1 ounce of the bark, boiled in a pint of water for twenty minutes, allowed to cool naturally, then strained.

• STRETCH MARKS •

Extra vitamin E, vitamin B3 and zinc, help to prevent stretch marks. A simple massage of ten drops of lavender oil and ten drops of neroli oil added to one tablespoonful of almond oil is helpful.

• OEDEMA (TISSUE SWELLING) •

I do not like to give herbs internally unless absolutely necessary during pregnancy. To treat oedema I prefer to prescribe hand or foot baths morning and evening. I recommend diuretic herbs like dandelion, hawthorn or broom. Ginger poultices applied over the kidneys daily are comforting and effective.

Oedema should be reported to your GP as it can be a warning sign of pre-eclampsia.

• VARICOSE VEINS •

A family history of low arterial blood pressure makes you more liable to varicose problems. Ten per cent of pregnant women will get varicose veins during the course of pregnancy. Veins in the legs are particularly prone. The problem is exacerbated by calcium deficiency, by standing for long periods, which impedes the circulation, and by wearing constricting clothes or shoes. Some authorities recommend making a strong decoction of oak bark tea and soaking cotton stockings in it. These should then be pulled up over the varicose veins and covered in plastic to prevent leaks. The stockings should be kept on all night.

Bioforce's hyperisan tincture taken internally is also helpful.

• HAEMORRHOIDS •

Haemorrhoids are tiny varicose veins just inside the anus. Alternating hot and cold sitz baths of oak bark tea are helpful, as are iced-cold poultices of non-alcoholic witch hazel applied externally around the anus. Some people suggest inserting a piece of potato about the size of the little finger into the rectum for instant relief. A junk food diet will make you more predisposed to haemorrhoids; yet another good reason to eat well.

• URINARY INFECTIONS •

You should inform your GP if you suspect you have a urinary tract infection. Initially treat this by drinking pints of home-made, unsweetened, cranberry juice. If this hasn't worked within twenty-four hours use liberal amounts of raw garlic in the diet. If the infection persists for more than a few days consult a professional medical herbalist who will need to choose appropriate herbs for you (some natural anti-infectives are contra-indicated in pregnancy).

• HIGH BLOOD PRESSURE •

During pregnancy you will have frequent checks for high blood pressure. I seldom have patients suffer from this if they work with me throughout their pregnancy on their diet, but if necessary you can increase your intake of raspberry leaf tea; garlic and hawthorn berry are excellent tonics. None of these will hurt you or the baby. Cayenne pepper mixed into juice will raise the blood pressure if it is too low and reduce it if it is too high. If the blood pressure is raised because of stress, meditation and visualisation will also help.

Inform your GP of any herbal preparations you are taking for high blood pressure.

• MUSCLE PAIN •

Some women get persistent shooting pains down their thighs during the last part of pregnancy, occasionally earlier. These pains can be caused by the baby pressing on the related nerves in the pelvis; during the last part of the pregnancy they are the result of the baby pressing its head against the cervix trying to soften it up and get ready for birth. Lie down and ask your partner to press the muscles inside your thighs and between your hip bones and pelvic bones. He will easily detect any tight muscles in these areas and should press them firmly and consistently until the tightness disappears. If you do not have a partner, ask a friend to press these muscles.

• PHLEBITIS (BLOOD CLOTS) •

Changes in sex hormones in pregnancy can cause the blood to clot more readily. Apply external compresses of ice-cold witch hazel. Raw onion rubbed over the area externally also helps, as does eating garlic.

• CONSTIPATION •

The extra progesterone produced during pregnancy tends to over-relax the intestinal muscles. A diet high in raw food with plenty of liquids including potassium broth, herbal teas, fruit smoothies, soups and nut milks will help, as will more exercise. The Intestinal Corrective Formulas 3 and 1 are both quite safe to take during pregnancy (pages 72 and 73).

• INDIGESTION •

The first steps to recovery from indigestion are food combining and chewing your food conscientiously. Even juices should be swished around the mouth and mixed with plenty of saliva before swallowing. Don't drink water with your meals, but potassium broth and freshly pressed juices are permissible. Make sure you eat little and often. Slippery elm gruel, digestive enzymes or the formulation on pp.188–9 will all help.

• BACKACHE •

If you get backache try the following exercises, adapted from yoga. The yogic tailor pose opens the legs wider than sitting cross-legged on the floor. The soles of the feet are placed together and held up as close to the groin as possible using both hands, allowing the knees to drop open. For the cat exercise, the woman kneels on the floor, with her arms straight from her shoulders. She should breathe in as she arches her back, lifting her spine towards the ceiling and letting her head fall between her arms. Next, she should breathe out as she curves her spine in the opposite direction, dropping her spine towards the floor. At this stage her head should be raised, as if she is looking at the ceiling. The movements should be repeated in a gentle, rocking manner. When you bend down always squat on the knees rather than bending from the hips and when you sit on the floor sit in the Indian fashion with your legs crossed at the ankle and your knees bent or adopt the yogic tailor pose. Both of these postures will tone up the birthing muscles. Birkenstock sandals help to relieve foot and back pain.

Hot and cold sitz baths will also alleviate back pain. You may find that a chiropractor or an osteopath will be able to help. Massage might help too.

Ensure you are getting plenty of calcium in the diet. Many of my patients have found the concentrated chlorophyll in sprouted wheatgrass juice helpful. Rubbing a drop of Olbas oil into the area of the pain may help. Pressing the sore spots firmly with the thumbs will also relieve much of the stress.

• MISCARRIAGE •

I have used a combination of three parts of false unicorn root and one part of lobelia many times with great success to avert a miscarriage. Use one teaspoonful of this combination to a cup of hot water to make a tea. Take half a cup every half hour. Once the bleeding has stopped take the tea every hour for the rest of the day and then three times a day for the next three days. The beauty of this combination of herbs is that they will not interfere with the natural process of miscarriage if the foetus is damaged or dead and needs expulsion. I always issue it to my pregnant patients so that they can have it on standby and so have peace of mind.

If you do suffer a miscarriage take Bach Rescue Remedy, available from all health stores.

• PRENATAL FORMULATION •

This has facilitated many comfortable, easy births. It is designed to elasticise the pelvic and vaginal areas, strengthening the reproductive organs for easier delivery. It should only be taken six weeks before the birth, **never sooner.** Take three size 0 capsules of the finely powdered herbs morning and evening with raspberry leaf or squawvine tea.

Equal parts of: *penny royal*
squawvine   *false unicorn*
blessed thistle   *raspberry leaves*
black cohosh   *lobelia*

I have never yet given this out to a pregnant woman who has not said that it has helped her to some degree during the birthing process.

• EASING DELIVERY •

It is best to use tinctures just before and during delivery as they are assimilated very quickly. One teaspoonful of tincture of black cohosh in water or juice as needed during labour will ensure a prompt delivery, and if uterine pushing is weakening give fifteen drops of goldenseal tincture every half hour. Many women fast before giving birth swearing that fasting enhances their performance by increasing their stamina and concentration. Others prefer to eat something high in carbohydrate at the first sign of labour.

The adrenal formula on p.172 will assist during the first stage of labour and will also help the baby, whose adrenal glands are now working hard. It may also be administered after the birth if the mother is exhausted. As an alternative administer cayenne pepper in juice. To alleviate shock use cayenne tincture mixed with apple cider vinegar and honey diluted with hot water. This also will warm you and give you energy.

• PAIN •

When I interviewed Diane Bjornson, an extremely experienced midwife who has delivered thousands of babies, she said that one of the most effective pain relievers for labour was to administer a lobelia enema just before labour began, or at least right at the very beginning. Other herbs which she found helpful included one teaspoonful of motherwort tincture taken as often as needed in something hot in early labour, and later on skullcap or St John's Wort for easing the pain.

• AFTER THE BIRTH •

For the pains of afterbirth (which some women may experience) use a tincture of St John's wort, massaged into the lower spine. Alternatively, ten drops can be taken orally, as needed. It is important to maintain natural calcium levels in the diet – carrot juice and rice bran syrup are good sources. Catnip, valerian, cayenne and lobelia mixed together in equal parts (20 drops at a time) in diluted grape juice and taken as often as required, can be of great help. Country leaf tea contains a cell proliferant which helps to rebuild the body. Yellow dock and dandelion root tea decocted, will help to boost the circulation of blood. The diet should be rich in raw vegetables and fruit.

CHAPTER 9:

MENOPAUSE AND BEYOND

––––

The Ancient Greeks used to call the menopause the Climacteric meaning 'a step in the ladder'. They saw it as simply one of the seven-year periods forming the life cycle. They understand it as a time when gradually, gently and gracefully a woman was relieved of the burden of being able to have children. Indeed, it is true that nature has designed the menopause to be a slow downward shift in the process of producing oestrogen output by the ovaries with minimal side-effects. In a healthy, well nourished, active woman the pituitary gland, which regulates hormone production in the body, signals the adrenal glands to increase their oestrogen output after the ovaries have ceased production and this back-up system helps to keep a small amount of oestrogen in the circulation, so maintaining a female body shape, female patterns of hair distribution and a female voice. If the adrenal glands are exhausted as the result of poor diet, constant stress, hypoglycaemia or any other nutritional deficiency the menopause may be difficult. Symptoms may include haemorrhaging, hot flushes and cold sweating, palpitations, vertigo, tingling, chills, nervousness, excitability, depression, irritability, fatigue, insomnia, headaches, muscle and bone aches and gastro-intestinal or urinary disturbances. The effects may include osteoporosis, a frequent desire to urinate or stress incontinence, the growth of unwanted body hair, the drying of vaginal secretions resulting in painful sex and vaginitis, weight gain, dry or itching skin and reduced breast size. None of these things need happen to you if you get yourself into really good shape well before the menopause starts.

Diet

During the menopause and as you continue to age the diet needs to be particularly good. Anything with chemicals in it should be rigorously avoided and, if you can manage, follow a vegan diet incorporating abundant portions of sprouted seeds, whole grains, royal jelly, pollen, bananas, carrots, potatoes, apples, cherries, plums and garlic, all of which are particularly rich in natural hormones. It is essential to ensure plenty of B and E vitamins as well as zinc and essential fatty acids in the diet. Foods rich in vitamin C and bioflavonoids are also important. As oestrogen levels in the body drop the capillary linings become thinner and leak more readily, hence hot flushes. Three to four citrus fruits with the white pith left on eaten daily will help hot flushes. Propolis, the sticky resin leaked by leaf buds and tree barks and consequently gathered by bees to cement their hives, is particularly rich in bioflavonoids. This is available in capsule form. For uncontaminated sources of propolis see Resources Directory.

• SUPERFOODS FOR THE MENOPAUSE •

VITAMIN E

Foods rich in vitamin E stimulate the production of oestrogen and help alleviate hot sweats. Vitamin E seems to exert a normalising effect on oestrogen levels. It has the ability to increase the hormone output in women who are deficient in it and lowers it in those who are prone to an excess.

Recommended foods: wholegrains and oils extracted from them, nuts and seeds.

VITAMIN B

Foods rich in the B-complex vitamins (such as nutritional yeast, wheat germ, whole grains and seed) enhance the effectiveness of oestrogenic hormones and help prevent menopausal arthritis as well as oedema. B-complex vitamins also boost the thyroid gland and as the whole endocrine system is intimately involved in menopausal changes this is important. A properly functioning thyroid gland is essential for normal sex hormone production because the thyroid secretes thyroxine, which has a direct stimulating effect on the sex glands. An underactive thyroid gland will lead to depleted sex glands and insufficient sex hormone output.

SEAWEEDS

All the seaweeds will help to improve the function of the thyroid gland and will help to some degree to control obesity if weight is a problem.

CALCIUM AND VITAMIN D

A malfunctioning parathyroid gland can upset calcium and vitamin D metabolism and eating foods rich in easily assimilable calcium is important to support parathyroid function. Vitamin D, besides improving mineral metabolism and utilisation is, of course, richly present in natural sunlight.

Recommended foods rich in calcium: tahini (sesame seed butter), nuts and seeds.

Foods rich in vitamin D: Spirulina, Chlorella. It is also made naturally by the body, when the skin is exposed to sunlight.

VITAMIN C AND BIOFLAVONOIDS

Foods rich in vitamin C and bioflavonoids act as detoxifiers, rejuvenators and stimulants of the thyroid and sex glands. Vitamin C also encourages the body to metabolise oestrogen and the bioflavonoids help hot flushes.

Recommended foods rich in vitamin C and bioflavonoids: abundant in raw vegetables and fruit. Bioflavonoids can be found in the white pith which surrounds citrus fruit.

ZINC

Zinc is necessary for reproductive hormone and enzyme production, for the formation of RNA and DNA, and for the proper utilisation of vitamins and minerals, especially for the metabolism of vitamin A and for the synthesis of insulin and protein.

Recommended foods rich in Zinc: Pumpkin and sunflower seeds.

All of these vitamins and minerals are particularly concentrated in spirulina, chlorella, nutritional yeast, whole grains, nuts and seeds and organic fruits and vegetables.

• HERBAL HELP •

There are many herbs rich in natural oestrogen-like substances which will help to smooth the transition from ovarian to adrenal production of oestrogen. These include wild yam, lady's slipper, passion flower, black cohosh, sarsaparilla, false unicorn, elder, licorice, fennel, Chinese angelica, sage, hops, Siberian ginseng, motherwort, marigold, false unicorn root and chaste tree.

I have had particular success helping women through any uncomfortable menopausal symptoms with the following formulation:

Hormone Replacement Therapy Tonic

Equal parts of the tinctures of: *chaste tree*
wild yam   *fennel*
    Chinese angelica

The dosage is normally forty drops morning and evening and after three months this can be reduced to twenty or thirty drops morning and evening.

This, coupled with the adrenal formulation on p.172, really helps maintain hormonal balance.

• HOT FLUSHES •

Most menopausal women experience hot flushes. It helps to wear layers of clothing so that you can peel a few off if a flush overwhelms you. Cool, but not cold, baths taken before bed are also useful.

• NIGHT SWEATS •

Sage helps alleviate or prevent night sweats. A very simple solution that I have found to work extremely well with my own patients is either three drops of essential oil of sage taken with a little honey in hot water just before bed, or fifteen drops of the tincture of sage taken three times a day. Dilute the tincture in a little water.

• EXCESSIVELY HEAVY PERIODS •

Normally, during menopause, there are longer and longer gaps between periods, which tend to become lighter and shorter until they eventually stop. Very occasionally, periods will stop suddenly once and for all, but this is rare.

It is never normal to have frequent heavy periods, or to pass blood clots during the menopause. If this happens to you consult your doctor immediately. Pain, spotting in between periods and after love making are equally unacceptable. In an emergency use cayenne as a douche (see p.44) I have also had great success using Bioforce's Tormentavena in tincture form. The dosage is normally fifteen drops three times a day before meals, but I emphasise again that if you are experiencing excessively heavy bleeding or bleeding between periods you must have a very thorough gynaecological check immediately.

• VAGINAL CHANGES •

The vagina sheds its epithelial cells continually. Harmless resident bacteria in the vagina help to decompose cell detritus and in doing so manufacture lactic acid which protects against harmful bacteria, but as oestrogen levels fall, the climate in the vagina changes dramatically. The cells of the lining thin and dry out and are unable to fend off invading bacteria. As a result offensive vaginal discharges are much more common during the menopause and afterwards. This in turn can cause pain on love making and not unnaturally put a women off sex altogether. Synthetic hormonal creams are not the answer. Such creams are easily absorbed into the bloodstream. Hormone replacement therapy is dangerous when administered in this way, orally or by transdermal patch (plasters containing HRT chemicals which are applied to the skin). In any case, it is not lack of oestrogen which makes vaginas dry. To put it simply, dryness is caused by underuse.

OVERCOMING DRYNESS

Regular sex, or masturbation if you don't have a partner or don't feel like sexual intercourse, keeps the vagina in good working order. Lubrication has much less to do with the intensity of stimulation than with its duration, so if you find yourself getting into difficulties share this information with your partner. However, experimenting must be done gently. In the post-menopausal woman the clitoris is relatively more exposed because of labial atrophy, so this sensitive area will become more vulnerable to direct stimulation through intercourse. Any very intense stimulation at this juncture, far from being exciting, can be distressing and painful. Saliva or KY jelly helps with vaginal lubrication as do foods rich in vitamin E, vaginal boluses made in a carrier base of coconut oil and slippery elm with generous additions of wheat germ oil, and vaginal douches of clay, made with four tablespoonfuls of clay to a litre of pure water.

If you do go off sex, don't feel a freak. It could be as much to do with the fact that your ageing partner is balding and has a paunch as with changes in you!

• INCONTINENCE •

Incontinence is a major problem in the West, but one which is hidden due to the fear of embarrassment. In fact, most women wet themselves from time to time and a survey of college students revealed that five per cent had said they leaked regularly, so this is not just a problem that comes with ageing. Incontinence may eventually become so severe that a woman has to wear absorbent pads to catch the urine which can escape at any time.

If incontinence is the primary problem, that is, it is not caused by a prolapse, surgical correction can be very unpredictable, and properly performed Kegal exercises are far more helpful (see p.92). All other exercise, especially yoga, will also strengthen and tone the muscles of the pelvic floor. If you know that your pelvic floor is weaker than it should be please act promptly and consult either a complementary practitioner or your GP.

Alternating hot and cold sitz baths are helpful as is the following formula:

Equal parts of:
parsley
juniper
marshmallow
gravel root

uva ursi
lobelia
ginger
black cohosh

Take two size 0 capsules three times a day with a cup of horsetail and parsley mixed in equal quantities to make a tea.

If incontinence is a problem during pregnancy omit the juniper and black cohosh from this formula.

• THE MYTH OF OSTEOPOROSIS •

Milk is touted as a great natural source of calcium, and we are told to eat plenty of calcium to prevent osteoporosis, or thinning of the bones. In fact, some evidence suggests that eating dairy products can increase the rate at which calcium is lost from the body and so hasten osteoporosis. As well as being high in calcium, dairy products are also high-protein foods. If you have too much protein in the diet, in milk products or from any other source such as meat, fish or eggs, the body has to get rid of the excess. To do this the kidneys lose calcium as they cleanse the blood of excess waste.

People in the United States and Scandinavian countries consume more dairy products than anywhere else in the world, yet they have the highest rate of osteoporosis. This fact emphasises the threat of excessive protein in the diet and supports the claim that dairy products offer no protection against osteoporosis.

The answer to osteoporosis, far from taking a diet rich in dairy products, is in essence to cut right down on your protein intake and preferably to become a vegan.

The body's ability to absorb and utilise calcium depends on the amount of phosphorus in the diet. The higher the calcium-phosphorus ratio, the less bone loss takes place and the stronger the skeleton, provided the intake of protein is not excessive. Fruit and vegetables contain high calcium-phosphorus levels.

HIGH RISK FACTORS FOR OSTEOPOROSIS

- A diet high in protein.
- Women who are light boned.
- Women who have subjected themselves to a lifetime of punishing diets.
- Women who don't take enough exercise. Weight-bearing exercise like brisk walking or jogging strengthens the bones. However, trained female athletes and excessive exercisers can sometimes stop their periods altogether and research has shown this is because they become oestrogen deficient. Unsurprisingly their bones start to suffer. So overexercise can be just as bad as underexercise. The recommended amount of weight-bearing exercise a week is forty minutes three or four times a week.
- Women who smoke. Smoking has been shown to force women into the menopause two years earlier than their non-smoking sisters because smoking depletes oestrogen in the body.
- There seems to be a genetic tendency to osteoporosis. For example, black women get osteoporosis far less than their white sisters.
- Women who only take a small amount of absorbable calcium into their diet. Note that caffeine and alcohol encourage the excretion of calcium as does excessive salt, which not only makes our bodies excrete more calcium but also encourages excretion of phosphorus, another important constituent of bone, so speeding up bone loss.
- Certain drugs increase the risk of osteoporosis including cortisone, thyroxine, tamoxifen, diuretics and antacids. If you are prescribed one of

these drugs, ask your doctor about the likely effects on your bone density.
● Women who have had total hysterectomies including removal of their ovaries have a much higher risk of osteoporosis.

IMPROVING THE ODDS AGAINST OSTEOPOROSIS

● Become a vegan or cut down your intake of animal protein.
● Cut out caffeine and cut right back on alcohol.
● Stop smoking.
● Ensure easily assimilable sources of calcium in the diet. Eat plenty of raw fruit and vegetables.
● Expose your skin to the healing rays of the sun for a short period each day – the actual length of time you spend in the sun will depend on your own skin type.
● Exercise regularly for forty minutes three or four times a week ensuring that it is weight-bearing exercise.
● Cut down on salt and eat a diet specifically rich in the superfoods indicated for the menopause (see pp.135–6).

• AGEING •

Since some of the normal processes of ageing become more noticeable at the same time as the menopause many women tend to confuse the two or even blame the menopause for accelerating ageing. In fact the first signs of ageing begin long before the menopause. From the age of ten onwards the lens of the eye begins to lose some of its elasticity and focus. Hearing loss also begins at the tender age of ten. The good news is that IQ and memory remain pretty much intact throughout life. We often envisage our brain as an ever-expanding sieve through which recent events and memories leak away but this is not in fact true. Creativity and intellectual flexibility depend on how much you summon them to use. Compare the brain to muscle; the old adage 'if you don't use it you lose it' applies to both. Your brain begins to shrink by about the age of twenty and by the time you reach forty you have already lost 20 gm of it. This loss continues at the rate of one gram a year for the rest of your life. But, we only ever employ ten per cent of our brain, so there is still room for continuing intellectual improvement and flexibility.

THE PROCESS OF AGEING

The body's ability to ward off wear and tear declines from the age of 40 and most women notice that it becomes much harder to lose weight. Only the face and the head continue to grow, their dimensions expand slightly for twenty more years. The weight of gravity pressing down on the body suppresses the spinal column and the intervertebral discs deteriorate leading to a decrease in height. Inverted yoga postures and slant boards help here. Cells tend not to regenerate as quickly in a forty-year-old body as they do in a younger one. Bones take longer to mend, cuts and bruises don't heal as rapidly and the heart loses its capacity to pump at a peak rate under exercise and stress.

Reserves throughout the body diminish. The thyroid shrinks, slowing down the metabolic rate (hence the difficulty in losing weight) and signals a subsequent decline in other hormones. The muscles and tissues that support the womb and bladder tend to stretch and loosen, the number of pubic and scalp hairs diminish and the upper lip and cheeks sprout hairs. Fatty tissue is lost from beneath the surface of the skin so the lines of expression whenever you smile, frown or look surprised become more deeply entrenched as the skin loses its elasticity. There is no going back. For women who have spent their whole youth being judged by their physical appearance the ageing process can leave an enormous lingering sense of loss.

THE BENEFITS OF AGEING

But there are great benefits to ageing. Would you like to repeat your teenage years? I wouldn't. Some benefits are the by-products of accomplishment, of seeing children grow up, of having done things that no one else will do in exactly the same way. Other benefits are the by-products of freedom, of not having to contend with the shifting hormonal tides or the crises of raising a family. Some of the most beautiful and fulfilled women I know are grandmothers.

Men somehow find it easier to accept women as leaders and heroines as they age. Georgia O'Keeffe, Margaret Mead, Simone de Beauvoir, Mother Teresa, Jane Brown, Margaret Thatcher, Mrs Ghandi – the roll call of honour is literally endless. It's a rare woman who would trade her mind and personality for her younger self's body. We are not getting older we are simply getting better because we are feeling better, more ourselves, less afraid.

• DIET, EXERCISE AND LONGEVITY •

Eat well for graceful ageing. Fasting slows down the ageing process (see p.55) as do the superfoods (see p.25). Exercise matters as much as ever it did. Extensive research going back to the 1950s proves that exercise does encourage longevity. A Harvard University study suggested that people who expended 2,000 calories a week exercising lived one to two years longer than their sedentary compatriots. But in order to work off 2,000 calories a week you will have to spend roughly one and a half years exercising, about the same amount of time gained lengthening your life!

THE BENEFITS OF EXERCISE

You can keep your exercise programme down to as little as 40 minutes four times a week and still protect yourself against circulatory problems and osteoporosis. Walking has the advantage of greatly reducing the risk of injury or sudden cardiac death through extreme and sudden overexertion. While our capacity to utilise oxygen diminishes with increasing age, it has been shown that a 60-year-old who exercises regularly can use oxygen as efficiently as a sedentary 40-year-old. The mere act of pumping the blood through the arteries helps to dislodge plaque from the arteries' walls and regular exercise helps regulate the levels of different types of fatty acid in the blood. Exercise also activates fibrinolysis, the body's natural anticlogging system of rapidly acting enzymes that immediately dissolve small abnormal clots before they are able to block the arteries.

Among its many other miraculous abilities the body is able to build new arteries which travel around any blockage and so protect the specific section in jeopardy. The only factor which will actually accelerate such development is exercise. During the menopause it is very common for the percentage of body fat to increase by as much as 11 lb (5.95 kg). Very gradually the total body weight tends to follow suit. Exercise can actually help to reverse this process.

Continuing mental alertness can be encouraged by the restorative tonic on p.151. Circulatory problems, including high blood pressure and angina, can be helped by the solutions on pages 162–3.

• MORAL SUPPORT •

My feeling is that friendships and love are even more important in old age than at any other time of life. Friendships have certainly been the balm and blessing of my own life and I anticipate that they will play an even more pivotal role as I grow older. And the secret of a happy and successful old age? A Russian man interviewed in extreme old age, and claiming to be 166 said 'I was never in a hurry with my life and I am in no hurry to die now. There are two sources of long life. One is a gift from nature, and the pure air and the clean water of the mountains, the fruit of the earth, peace, rest and the soft warm climate of the highlands. The second source is within us. He lives long who enjoys life and who bears no jealousy of others, who's heart harbours no malice or anger, who sings a lot and cries a little, who rises and retires with the sun, who likes to work and who knows how to rest.'

PART THREE

TROUBLE SHOOTING

Mental pressures
Physical pressures
Holistic herbal first aid

CHAPTER 10:

MENTAL PRESSURES

———

• THE MIND-BODY CONNECTION •

There has been a very exciting revolution going on in medicine over the last two decades. More and more research confirms the intimate connection of the mind and the body. The way our mind works controls the way our body works. Of course, the control goes both ways and body chemicals give feedback to the mind via the brain. Aberrations in this mind/body connection are one of the major strands in the intricate weave of factors that cause illnesses. Scientists who study the new science of psychoneuroimmunology are discovering what naturopaths have known for thousands of years; that everything is connected to everything else in the body. I believe that at some point they are going to find everything in and around the human body is part of an entire field in which there is a myriad of relationships between all the parts. Let me explain, starting with a discussion of personal responsibility. My beliefs might seem strange to some, but try to read them without prejudice.

PERSONAL RESPONSIBILITY

Many beliefs we have about ourselves are formed in our earliest years. The belief that we are not solely responsible for ourselves is one of the most enduring, and this is precisely the case for children. When we were children many things were beyond our control. Our twentieth-century concept of childhood is that it is a time of diminished responsibility reinforced with a comforting knowledge that there is somebody more powerful to step in and provide a solution. Problems begin when we carry childhood beliefs into adulthood. As adults, so many of us cling to the belief that things are beyond our control because the prospect of being totally responsible for ourselves is very frightening. I believe the depth of this fear can be so great that we actually give ourselves life-threatening diseases rather than accept personal responsibility.

It is fairly common for people who won't accept that they are their own final arbitrator to use disease as an excuse for relinquishing personal responsibility, although it is extremely rare for such people to acknowledge that this is what they are doing. It is far less common to find people who revel in the power that they have over their own lives and who live to fulfil their dreams. They rarely suffer chronic disease, although occasionally they may become victims of an acute but transient complaint as the result of environmental hazards, injury or infection.

DRIVER MESSAGES

Driver messages are often the hardest to shake off. These are messages given to their children by parents wanting to make those children successful in life. The children see their success as being socially desirable so accept such messages as being given in their own best interest. The child is coerced by fear into following driver messages. Parental disapproval for not following such messages is seen as a threat to her own existence because the child feels she is only loved as long as she is top of the class, speedy, strong, etc. Failing to fulfil such parental directives means the child puts herself at risk of losing love and support; to a helplessly young child this feels, quite literally, life threatening. Driver messages can lead to a lot of anguish as the child grows up struggling to maintain an adult lifestyle based upon her childish beliefs.

Driver messages and illness

Once genetic and constitutional factors, environmental hazards, age, lifestyle, and other variables are taken into account, it can be seen that a strong 'be perfect' driver message may contribute to a stroke in one person or to a brain tumour in another. The actual outcome depends on the degree of acceptability of certain diseases within family and community circles. Diseases, like table manners, are modelled on adults. If the disease which actually develops as a result of a driver message becomes sufficiently distressing the discomfort caused may motivate the person to face the fear of, and then break away from, that childhood belief. Once a woman has decided to become well for herself and not simply to suppress the discomfort, she will no longer need to use the illness as a mental prop, and from this state of joyful self-responsibility she can then move towards attaining good health.

I hope I have persuaded you that illness is the physical and psychological result of a cocktail of driver messages and cultural beliefs which is fed to us from before birth. Of course external factors contribute too, including genetics, the manner of your birth, environmental hazards, exercise, diet, etc. Admittedly not all of these are under our control, but we can choose to use them to push us into being ill or not.

If you accept my argument, it is obvious that we should all be looking at undoing our programming and empowering ourselves with affirmations which encourage and allow us to be what we want to be and not to model ourselves on our parents' aspirations for us. Rest easy. If the damage has already been done it is not irrevocable. **It is possible to change things**.

• SELF-LOVE AND CHANGING •

There is a healing force present inside each one of us which mirrors the illness force. If you acknowledge a large proportion of your illness as self caused, you can then work on putting that portion into self-healing. By starting with the premise that a large proportion of your illness is of your own making you come to the inescapable conclusion that you can actively choose to do something about it. This recognition lets you become responsible for yourself and puts you in control of your own healing.

TAKING RESPONSIBILITY FOR YOUR PAST

Before you can take responsibility for the future you must take account of the past. Firstly, you need to accept that your actions were always your own. Once you accept responsibility for the old hurts you drop their burdensome weight and abandon the anger that still echoes around them. You must come to accept that you must change the way you were in order to survive. Once you have changed, you can always reverse the process and change back if that is what you need to do in order to survive in the future.

BEING ILL

The simple tools you need to bring about change are self-approval and self-acceptance. Given that you created the illness and invested in it, however subconsciously, you have the power to get rid of it. Illness alone is impotent. I know I only ever give myself a cold in order to give myself permission to stop work. Fate doesn't simply point her finger at me and visit a cold on me. I believe a stroke is not something that happens to a person by chance. It is something they choose to have when they are pushed to their furthest limit and are too scared to live. My feeling is we don't die, we kill ourselves. Sometimes being ill is the best way we know of getting what we want. Health involves a willingness to take the responsibility for the decision to be ill.

Illness is an invaluable learning process. All things being equal we deliberately give ourselves an illness in order to take care of our more debilitating physiological needs. By dulling pain with chemicals or by cutting out diseased tissue with surgery we merely remove something that was taking care of us. If you absorb this revolutionary idea you can learn from your illness. I believe cure is only possible if we accept this belief and then choose options other than the illness option. Those of you who are outward bound on a course of self-discovery and self-responsibility will gain little from allopathic methods. Chemicals merely dull the physical and psychological symptoms, thereby decreasing rather than increasing awareness of the problem.

BEING AFRAID

I believe that fear is the basis of all illness. If a person who has just had a stroke is offered the option of surviving by confronting her greatest fear, she will often astonish me by choosing the stroke. She needs her disease in order to avoid fear. It is a fear which has its roots in childhood beliefs. The woman is too afraid to take responsibility for herself.

We are, all of us, afraid. Afraid of not living fully, of being hurt, of death, of loneliness, of losing the securities we have, of not being loved. Normally what we do with fear is invent belief systems to try to make it go away. But fear is insidiously pervasive. We tend to treat fear as an external thing, as if it was something outside of us that has come in and taken over. But the reality of it is that when there is fear we are fear. It is not that we are having fear, fear is us. Fear freezes actions. Where there is fear there cannot be any learning. Fear and learning are incompatible bed fellows. But fear, properly handled, is a great psychological teacher. To watch it, to attend to it, is to learn about yourself. Consider fear the opener of many doors. Experiencing our fear, living it so that the fear is us, empowers us, changing our awareness. And it is self-awareness we need in order to accept ourselves, whoever, wherever and however we are.

SELF-LOVE

The truest beauty any woman can have is the beauty of spirit triumphant. The greatest and most enduring love is self-love. Be kind, firm and funny to yourself before it's too late. Self-responsibility and self-esteem are fundamental requirements for health and happiness.

All problems stem from one basic problem, lack of self-love. Bad relationships, stifled creativity and physical disease all have their origin in lack of self-love. Our thoughts determine our emotional reactions and these in turn have a profound affect on our physical health, our level of satisfaction, our work and the quality of our relationships.

In loving ourselves as profoundly, unconditionally and deeply as we would our truest lover we find the power that will heal us. Self-love dissolves anger, fear and resentment. It changes damaging thought patterns, resentment, criticism, guilt, fear and outmoded ideas that do not nourish and support us into positive attributes.

• THEORY INTO PRACTICE •

When you step onto this path of self-growth, of change, of loving and supporting yourself, it really doesn't matter where you start. You could begin with the cleansing techniques outlined in Chapter 4; they will inevitably lead you on to even better things. Or you could begin with the mind and the spirit which will lead you back to the body. Mind and body are all one. When you begin the process of transforming your life you find everything is transformed. It is a bit like house cleaning. It doesn't matter where you begin, the important thing is to keep going and eventually the whole house will sparkle and shine.

I often tell my patients: whatever the question is, love is the answer. There is no better way to become yourself, no better way to save yourself, no better way to heal yourself than love.

I will now discuss how self-love can transform a range of common problems.

• **DEPRESSION** •

PSYCHOLOGICAL CAUSES

Statistics show that women suffer more mental health problems than men. The mentally ill occupy one third of British hospital beds; the majority of these are taken by women, and women are the largest users of tranquilisers.

Wellbeing is the result of feeling in control of immediate life situations, being free from anxiety and having feelings of accomplishment of being in good health and having lots of energy. Depression stems from **not** being in control of one's life. Depression comes as the result of oppression. It affects women particularly badly because many women depend upon their partners for their income, or rely on welfare or social security payments or low-paid jobs. Men's salaries are still higher than women's. There are still very few women who are completely financially independent in spite of the fact that now more than two-thirds of women work outside the home. As women grow older they become increasingly more dependent on their children, if not for money for transportation, companionship or nursing when they are ill.

Pauline Bart, a feminist psychologist, defines depression as the response to powerlessness. She has compared women's passivity, fatigue and depression to the reaction of experimental animals who were given electric shocks no matter what they did. I loathe this kind of experimentation and certainly don't condone it, but the animals in the experiment behaved in ways similar to the way people in depression behave. They did not learn, they were passive, they did not eat, they did not even move much. When Pauline Bart studied middle-aged depressed women, she found that they were over involved with or overprotective of their children not because they wanted it that way, but because society forced on them the limited roles of wife and mother. When they lost either of these roles they responded with a loss of identity and with powerlessness and uselessness. Bart argues that society sets women up for depression by encouraging them, sometimes even forcing them, to put all 'all their eggs in one or at the most two baskets – the mother role and the wife role'.

Certainly women are more likely to suffer from depression if they are isolated, have no close friends to confide in, have no work outside the home, live in poor housing, have difficulty financially, look after toddlers at home full time or lose their own mother at an early age. Depression, of course, can apply equally to career women crippling themselves in the attempt to be superwomen. Those who retire unwillingly are notoriously prone to depression.

Of course, men have always known the price of success. Thousands of executives have paid for their jobs with blood money including ulcers, heart attacks and high blood pressure. Others have had to live with broken marriages, estranged children or their own addictions to tobacco, alcohol, drugs or work.

I look around me and I see that women are trying to change that pattern and hang on to their success together with their humanity. Feminist writer and activist Gloria Steinem contends that women aren't any more moral than men, they just haven't been offered their bite of the apple. But the women I know have watched what has happened to men who bit the apple, and have tried to learn from it. They may be carrying attaché cases and whipping out their gold cards but they don't want to be men, they only want to enjoy some of the privileges that men have enjoyed. They want an equal chance to succeed and an equal chance to fail. They want to be able to make their own mistakes as freely as men have. The cost of reaching for success may be high, but the cost of not reaching for success may be even higher.

Speaking up and standing up for yourself also helps beat depression. If your rights or dignity are being trampled on summon the energy to stand up for yourself. Say what you mean, show your feelings. Engage in purposeful activity. Make sure it is something you enjoy that will give you a sense of accomplishment. Don't hesitate to seek counselling if you feel it might be worth exploring. Valenarium zinicum (40 drops, three times daily) which are available from Bioforce can be helpful, as can Bach Flower remedies.

PHYSICAL CAUSES

Physical causes of depression include an underactive thyroid, nutritional deficiencies, heavy metal toxicity, food intolerances, hypoglycaemia, candidiasis and endocrine imbalance. Please get these all checked out. If your depression is extremely severe seek immediate medical help without hesitation. This doesn't necessarily mean to say you have to have drugs. I have seen acupuncture, biodynamics and nursing in anthroposophical hospitals work extremely well, none of which involves chemical medicines (see Resources Directory).

I have never found that herbs specifically help to alleviate depression but restoring good health is essential. I know that physical exercise helps, partly because it leads to chemical reactions which boost the nervous system. One of the most common signs of depression is fatigue and inertia. Make your exercise regular and enjoyable and, given time, it will revolutionise your physical and mental wellbeing.

• ANXIETY AND STRESS •

Adrenalin the hormone which prepares the body for 'fight or flight', is released during stress, raising blood pressure, tensing muscles, dilating pupils, speeding the heart rate and slowing down digestion. Too much stress, in other words too much adrenalin, chips away insidiously at an otherwise healthy body. In fact, stress had been implicated in a huge range of diseases including rheumatoid arthritis, hyperthyroidism, ulcerative colitis, heart attacks, strokes, cancer, and peptic ulcers. These seem to be afflicting women at nearly the same rate as men – a situation which has been ongoing since the late 1960s when women entered the competitive job market alongside men. Stress also influences the female hormones, for example it can contribute to a difficult menopause.

PHYSICAL SYMPTOMS

Physical symptoms of stress include fatigue and muscular weakness, sweating, trembling, breathlessness, choking, fainting, hypertension, palpitations, digestive upsets, over dependence on alcohol, drugs or tobacco, loss of interest in sex, insomnia, pins and needles anywhere in the body, or simply a succession of mysterious aches, pains and niggling discomforts. While allopathic medicine issues prescriptions that merely mask the symptoms and do nothing to deal with the social, emotional and physical conditions which are the cause, herbal medicine sees the nervous system holistically as an intrinsic part of the whole body's functions.

THE MIND AS A HEALING TOOL

As herbalists we feel that stress, neuroses, phobias, depression and even some psychotic illnesses can be greatly helped by using herbs which act as nervous restoratives and relaxants. Recognising the problem on a holistic level we also welcome counselling, encourage a good diet and plenty of exercise, and use stress management techniques such as meditation, yoga, self-hypnosis, visualisation, autogenics and biofeedback. All of these methods teach a person how to use the mind as a powerful healing tool. Some of them have been available to us for thousands of years.

Basic instruction in any of these methods of relaxation merely requires a good teacher, a comfortable room, time and willingness to undertake the training. It will cost you time and money but what you will gain is dexterity in manipulating the buttons and levers in the command control centre of your body – your mind. You will learn how to focus your mind on the physical body. You will learn a better way to control your physical body. Nurturing and dwelling on correct images and attitudes from moment to moment and day to day keep the body running smoothly. In a smoothly running body, hormones remain balanced and the immune system works efficiently. A body that enjoys this type of balance swings towards healing rather than illness. For details about organisations that will assist you with any of these relaxation techniques see Resources Directory.

HERBAL HELP

Herbs that will help to restore the tone of nerve tissue need to be taken over many months as they work slowly and deeply, but surely. They include oats, St John's wort, vervain, Siberian and Korean ginsengs, rosemary, skullcap, lavender and gota kola. My own nerve restorative formulation consists of:

Two parts: *St John's wort*
skullcap   *gota kola*
One part: *(All in tincture form)*
oat seed

This nourishes the nervous system and acts as a restorative tonic, particularly where the nervous system feels very depleted. In extreme cases I will often administer thirty drops in a little hot water every two to three hours.

Certain essential oils also have a beneficial action on the nervous system. A nerve tonic can be made by mixing two drops of neroli and two drops of melissa to four teaspoonfuls of almond oil. This should be rubbed into the chest and abdomen. Neroli and melissa, two drops of each, can be added to a tepid bath at night.

NB – If you are on any kind of chemical drugs for any mental disorder please ask your doctor to explain any possible side-effects, including possible addiction. You might be better to wean yourself off the drugs, under strict supervision, and to start on a course of holistic healing.

• INSOMNIA •

PHYSICAL CAUSES

Observe the advice on page 190. In addition cut out caffeine, salt and nicotine, because all of these can affect your sleeping pattern. Overeating before bed can make sleep difficult so try to eat larger meals during the day.

Nutritional deficiencies, particularly of the B-complex vitamins and calcium, are common factors in insomnia. Allergic reactions to food additives, colourings, preservatives and pesticides may cause an abnormally rapid heart rate (tachycardia) which does not allow the body to relax. A night-cap of alcohol is not a terribly good idea either as alcohol is a stimulant. One of the main causes of insomnia is going to bed at erratic times. I have particularly noticed this amongst air crew I have treated. Their odd working hours leave very many of them stressed, fatigued and sleepless. The important thing is to follow your own body rhythms and sleep regularly at a time that is comfortable for you. Don't worry if that is well after midnight. Six hours of refreshing sleep as part of a regular sleep schedule is much better than lying awake tossing and turning. Exercise is also terribly important. Remember also that sleep problems can often be connected with various drugs (see Appendix 1).

PSYCHOLOGICAL CAUSES

These are usually anxiety and depression. When depressed, it is common to wake in the early hours of the morning. Anxiety can often prevent sleep.

HERBAL HELP

Herbs can help, both taken through the skin and in herbal teas. Try hot foot baths; as these draw blood away from the head they make sleep easier. If you want to add infusions to your bath water, catnip, chamomile, lavender, lime blossom, woodruff and vervain all work particularly well either in warm bath water or in hot foot baths. Try tepid baths with lavender or chamomile oil added. Take a brief cold bath as a daily tonic. The wet sock treatment might help (see page 190).

Herbal Teas

If you want to experiment with herbal teas, try any of the following:

- lavender
- lemon balm
- lime flower
- passion flower
- skullcap
- valerian

Lavender tea should be drunk sparingly, no more than two cups a day. A single drop massaged into either temple can be helpful, but no more. Excessive use can cause convulsions in susceptible people. Lemon balm tea is delicious but needs to be made from fresh leaves. The dried leaves are a dusty, flavourless disappointment. If using lime flowers, ensure that your sources are fresh, as ageing flowers can be poisonous. Skullcap tea placed in a flask beside the bed is particularly helpful for those who wake up suddenly in the night full of unnamed fears and premonitions of calamity; it can be especially helpful if you add the Bach Flower remedies, aspen and walnut.

Valerian taken as a decoction tends to depress the nervous system and can cause depression and headaches in large doses. It is not one of my favourite teas because it tastes horrid. There are some who find it unexpectedly stimulating because their digestive enzymes are unable to transform valerian oil into the calming principle, valerianic acid. I prefer to use it in foot baths but if you do want to try a tea, use the fresh root covered with one pint (600 ml) of freshly boiled **but not boiling** hot water and allow it to cool and steep for twenty-four hours. Making it a decoction with prolonged heat dissipates the essential oils, which are the principal healing ingredients. Sixty drops of passion flower tincture taken three-quarters of an hour before bedtime works particularly well for those unfortunate enough to experience bad menopausal symptoms.

Of course please don't neglect those invaluable tools, relaxation exercises, autogenics and biofeedback.

• NIGHTMARES •

Most dreams last between ten and thirty minutes and in an average night a woman will have four or five dreams. Women often dream about being indoors or in familiar settings. Their dreams tend to be peopled with more women than men and their themes are often friendly, with little overt sex. The faces they see are often recognisable. Men, on the other hand, confront strangers in dream scenes that are filled with physical violence. In their dreams male figures out-number female, but when a woman enters a male dream the physical activity may turn to sex.

PRE-MENSTRUAL DREAMS

Your hormonal cycle will affect your dreams. During the days immediately preceding menstruation, a woman's dreams can become charged with emotions. Women who dream at this time find dream themes becoming less friendly and their dream encounters becoming marred by anxiety and frustration. Dreams will often take on overtures of inadequacy and hostility.

During pregnancy, women often dream about large babies or litters of babies. To soothe any apprehension of having to deliver an impossibly large baby the dreams often come up with magical solutions. Interestingly, the woman's partner tends to disappear from her dreams in pregnancy and is replaced by her own mother.

USEFUL TREATMENTS

I have found the Bach Flower remedies particularly useful for nightmares, particularly aspen. Hydrotherapy can also be helpful. If the nightmares are associated with the menstrual cycle, the pre-crash tincture on page 113 often helps.

• DIFFICULTY IN ACHIEVING ORGASM •

For a woman, orgasm, emotion and moods come in a package and this is part of the reason why women have more difficulty than men climaxing in each and every sexual encounter. Of course, most of you already know this, intuitively understanding that conditions have to be right and that your lover has to take account of your needs if you are to have an orgasm. Most women find it acceptable to remain at the plateau arousal phase (the stage before orgasm) from time to time, but when this happens too often, or all the time, it causes both physical and emotional problems for the woman and for the relationship.

The single most common cause for a woman failing to achieve orgasm is inadequate stimulation. Often the man gets blamed, verbally or silently, for ejaculating too soon. But just as often it is not really his fault and a woman must share some of the responsibility for bringing herself to orgasm. She has to give directions in her own way, and to do this she has to feel free to speak up, say what feels good, change positions, move a man's hand (or her own) down to her vulva and teach him how to stimulate her entire genital area the way she is used to having it stimulated through her own masturbatory experience.

CAUSES

In most cases, difficulty in achieving orgasm is attributable to psychological rather than physical disorders. There are a couple of conditions which are physical but apart from these, any source of sexual dysfunction stems from a woman's thoughts and feelings about the act itself and about the man she is with.

Dyspareunia is the technical term for painful sexual intercourse often because of a lack of natural lubrication in the vagina. Without this natural lubrication penetration causes too much friction. Instead of pleasurable sensations, the sensory nerves in the labia and the vagina send messages to the brain that are interpreted as pain. Similar pain messages can be caused by pelvic infection or an abnormal growth in the uterus.

APHRODISIAC

Herbal pharmacopoeias through the ages have contained lots of aphrodisiacs and some of them do have a mildly helpful effect including damiana, saw palmetto, cola, cinnamon and cocoa beans. However, the most reliable aphrodisiac of all is a woman's mind.

• EATING DISORDERS AND BODY IMAGE •

Women and men have always lied to each other through images. Many women spend their lives measuring themselves against idealised images, and if there is any discrepancy they leap to the conclusion that they have failed, not that the images were false. Pain, self-hatred and envy all follow. One of the reasons for the success of the Women's Movement was that it questioned idealised images of femininity. Of course, the Movement gave rise to new images, some of them as stereotyped as the old, but at least the women thus represented were exciting and competent.

THE 'IDEAL' IMAGE

Almost all the images we have of ourselves have been given to us by men. No wonder they cause us so much pain and discomfort! A man's version of femininity is all about how women are held back, held in, possibly for ever. So women grow up learning to be dainty. We do not gorge ourselves on food (at least when anyone is looking) and we don't swear. We are destined to be as neat as a pin, as fresh as a daisy, modest and entirely obliging. A feminine woman is not supposed to have moods, dark fears, fierce desires or beliefs. She is not supposed to enjoy solitude or anything else that would interfere with her responsiveness to others. The core of her orientation is to please and to soothe. Femininity entails a lot of waiting to be chosen. It was Marilyn Monroe who observed 'Being a sex symbol is a heavy load to carry, especially when one is tired, hurt and bewildered'.

Behind femininity is a terror of being alone. Young girls are taught the feminine woman will attract a man, the non-feminine one won't. So we grow up yanking our hair around rollers that stab the scalp; plucking sensitive eyebrows; pouring hot wax over skin to rip the hairs out. Some of us break our noses and have them reset, or have our skin sanded. Some women have pouches under their eyes slit out. Sagging chins are cut out and thrown away. And we think Chinese foot binding was barbaric?! This, then, is the female experience and it is absolutely crazy. We are not judged by what we can do, but by how we look. And the judges are men. No wonder so many women have problems with body image.

Those of us who no longer want to use men's eyes as our score cards are using and appreciating our bodies in totally new ways. Our legs are there to carry us, they do not need to be slim, to be shaved or to be waxed. We should celebrate muscle, sinew and powerful flesh. Women are seen in the business world as directors, astronauts, athletes, telephone engineers, carpenters, plumbers, electricians, publishers – doing anything, doing everything. However, there are still too many of us starving ourselves to death, vomiting secretly, mutilating ourselves for the benefit of men.

• ANOREXIA AND BULIMIA •

In general anorexics are fixated with avoiding food and having exercise. They are often hyperactive and suffer bouts of depression. Bulimics swing between uncontrollable eating binges and self-induced vomiting. The current medical approach is one of force-feeding and counselling. It is interesting to note that a zinc deficiency is common to both illnesses, also that biochemical disturbance can often be brought on by periods of crash dieting on fewer than 1,200 calories a day.

Anorexia can bring on bulimia as can foods that affect blood sugar levels (particularly those which contain refined sugar). Some recent research suggests that vitamin B3 deficiency may precipitate anorexia. There is now substantial research which suggests that anorexia is due to a **combined** deficiency of zinc and essential fatty acids, and indeed the two do work synergistically. Eating disorders can start after pregnancy, so a folic acid deficiency may be indicated.

HERBAL HELP

A herbalist will treat anorexics with bitter herbs to stimulate the liver and relaxants to strengthen the nervous system. These need to be individually prescribed although some have had great success with Marsdenia condurango. Bulimia is often treated by prescribing a nutrient rich diet, supplemented with B-complex vitamins and vitamin C.

For any eating disorders my advice would be to search out the help of a naturopath or medical herbalist with an extremely sound knowledge of nutrition and counselling.

• AGORAPHOBIA AND CLAUSTROPHOBIA •

Agoraphobia or fear of open spaces can be understood as a biochemical imbalance, and at the Department of Molecular Biology at the University of Pennsylvania it has been very successfully treated by taking two tablespoonfuls of linseed oil with each meal. The linseed oil used on wooden items is not for internal consumption. For the correct source see Resources Directory. Both agoraphobia and claustrophobia, a dread of being confined in enclosed rooms or small spaces, can also be the result of an early traumatic experience. Counselling is certainly indicated.

• HYPERVENTILATION •

This simply means over breathing; that is breathing in excess of physiological requirements. Normally air is drawn into the lungs where oxygen is absorbed into the blood whilst carbon dioxide is given off as a waste product. Carbon dioxide dissolved in the blood causes the blood acidity to rise. The kidneys and the lungs are both involved in regulating blood acidity, the kidneys by selective extraction and the lungs by blowing off excess carbon dioxide when we breathe out. Buffer chemicals in the blood are able to mop up some excess acidic and alkaline ions but there is a limit to how much compensation can take place this way, particularly when something is causing a chronic departure from the optimum acidity.

Hyperventilation lowers the carbon dioxide levels excessively which depletes blood bicarbonate and upset the body's entire acid-based equilibrium causing symptoms in susceptible patients. The failure to breathe properly, resulting in oxygen starvation for both the body and the brain, is surprisingly common. The two most typical symptoms are chronic fatigue and dizziness.

DIAGNOSIS AND TREATMENT

Diagnosis of hyperventilation and failure to breathe are difficult. But as problems are partly exacerbated by a nervous system gone awry, a skilled medical herbalist will make good use of nervines which restore and relax. I have had success with this strategy, coupled with sending the patient to yoga classes to learn correct breathing. Acupuncture can also be helpful.

> *It is important to consult a well qualified, experienced therapist, because of the difficulty in making a diagnosis.*

TOP HERBS FOR ALL ROUND MENTAL HEALTH:

- **Antispasmodic herbs**   Lobelia, black Cohosh root;
- **Nerve food herbs**   Skullcap herb, oat meal, seeds and straw;
- **Painkillers**   Feverfew leaves, wild lettuce leaves, seeds and juice;
- **Sedative/nervine herbs**   Valerian root, hops flowers, wood betony leaves, passion flower leaves, blue vervain root and herb, chamomile leaves and flowers, lime leaves and flowers, feverfew leaves.

CHAPTER 11:

PHYSICAL PRESSURES

• ALLERGIES •

Given the fact that we are now ingesting so many chemicals in our food and breathing in so many poisons from our environment it is not surprising that scientific literature is bulging with information about the so called allergic response. We are told to avoid allergy triggers, whether they be animals, pollens, house mites, foods, chemicals or artificial flavourings and colourings. Despite all this, I don't actually subscribe to the theory of allergies. Let me explain why.

MAXIMISING LIVER HEALTH

An allergy is first registered in the liver or by the parasympathetic nervous system. When your body comes into contact with a substance to which it is intolerant it immediately releases specific chemicals, including histamine. Its response is carried to every part of the body by the bloodstream and although you may suffer only localised symptoms like diarrhoea, streaming eyes or an itchy skin, every part of you will be affected.

The tenth cranial nerve, the vagus nerve, is a major player in the intolerance response. Beginning at the base of the brain it branches through both the eye and ear zones and sinuses, travelling on down to the neck and throat and across the bronchial tree and lungs and then into the stomach and pancreas. Any of these areas can be affected by a substance to which you appear intolerant.

In many cultures anger is believed to reside in the liver or the gall-bladder. This is not by any means as odd as it sounds. After all, the emotions we feel have a basis in biochemistry. When we feel angry a complex mixture of hormones and other chemicals rushes to various parts of the body readying us for action. One of the important functions of the liver is its role in transforming and removing excess hormones from the blood. When it is diseased or overburdened its ability to do this is impaired. I would estimate that more than half of the patients I work with who suffer metabolic shock or a disturbance of the liver function are more generally sick because of their thoughts and emotions, not simply as a result of poor diet or inadequate levels of nutrition. Your liver bears the brunt of unexpressed and suppressed emotions more than any other part of the body. You can only ever be really healthy if your liver is allowed the freedom to practise its alchemy uninterrupted. I believe that the body's chemical balance mechanisms are upset more profoundly by shock, grief, jealousy, greed, resentment, fear, depression, possessiveness, lack of self-esteem and anger than they are by the odd cream cake, glass of champagne or even meat!

Of course, life is made much harder for your long-suffering liver if you put man-made chemical rubbish into your body in combinations that are so new evolution has not provided mechanisms to break them down. So-called allergy responses occur when the liver is presented with such new chemical combinations or emotional suppression occurs. A healthy liver in an emotionally happy body, enjoying good overall balance, will be able to minimise any responses to allergies, even to less than perfect foods and various types of pollutions.

So I believe we should be maximising liver health rather than burdening ourselves with long lists of restrictions. Some enlightened clinical ecologists are beginning to wake up to the fact that allergy triggers are primarily emotional. In other words it might not be fish you are allergic to, it might be that your body is responding to the memory that your mother cuffed you round the ear every time you sat in front of a piece refusing to eat it.

In my own practice I have found over and over again that allergies respond faster, more completely and more permanently once a person's emotions are sorted out and they have detoxified, than they do to all manner of restricted diets or complex desensitising programmes. A generous portion of emotional contentment, the honest ability to talk about and deal with all those bitter grievances, a diet using foods that are in season, free, as far as possible, of chemicals, kidney and liver flushes, liver tonic herbs and spring tonics in season, unimpeded circulation, and a bowel that works freely should be enough to keep you out of an allergist's office.

See page 95 for kidney flush and page 63 for liver flushes, and liver tonic herbs. Spring tonics are traditionally taken in the spring to clean out the impurities which may have accumulated in the liver as a result of an overly rich, winter diet and to purify the blood. The herbs most commonly used include dandelion and burdock. Alternatives include chicory root (roasted), chickweed and yellow dock.

• HYPERACTIVITY •

The causes of hyperactivity are legion. Food allergy is a major contributive factor as are chemical exposure, nutrient deficiencies, hypoglycaemia, candida, parasitic infection, heavy metal toxicity, antenatal lack of oxygen, excessive alcohol consumption or an intolerance to alcohol, smoking, underlying physical illness, a bad reaction to drugs, and environmental lighting and radiation.

DIAGNOSIS AND TREATMENT

The first thing you need to do is to make certain that there is no underlying medical condition; then you should get tested for food intolerances. This can be done by a clinical ecologist, a Vega tester, an acupuncturist experienced with reading pulses to test food intolerance, or an iridologist. Foods to which you are intolerant then need to be excluded from your daily regime.

If this is not the complete answer also add vigorous exercise to your daily programme (this should be worked out in advance with a professional), stop watching television and use Turkish Baths or saunas twice a week. Have a massage along the spine using an infusion of poppy petals and take foot baths of chamomile or lime blossom morning and evening.

• HIGH BLOOD PRESSURE •

Let me begin by saying that **high blood pressure is not a disease**. It is simply a defensive and corrective measure, a means of dealing with pathological conditions such as toxaemia (overall poisoning of the body as the result of the failure to remove toxic waste through the eliminative channels), glandular disturbances, defective calcium metabolism, malfunctioning kidneys, degenerative changes in the arteries, obesity and emotionally caused physical dysfunction. Often high blood pressure has no obvious medical cause at all yet there are hundreds of thousands of people who take blood pressure drugs every day, assuming they will need them for the rest of their lives. To my mind it is a complete waste of time lowering the blood pressure unless the cause of the condition can be removed. An iridology test will often get to the heart of the problem. For further details on the damage that chemical drugs to treat blood pressure do, see Appendix 1: Some chemical drugs which give cause for thought.

Average blood pressure reads 120/80. It is the lower figure, called the diastolic reading, which is the more important because this records the rebounding of blood back through the arteries and the pressure they are under even at rest. The vast majority of hypertensive people can be helped by a simple naturopathic approach; however, it does require dedication and persistence from the patient.

FASTING

I have found a supervised juice fast lasting for three to four weeks is an excellent way of bringing the blood pressure down to normal, and it certainly produces a very rapid reduction in the systolic pressure (which records how the blood bounds outwards from the heart through the arteries). The juices I use are citrus, blackcurrant, grape, carrot or spinach. Vegetable juices can be spiced with a dash of onion or garlic. A brown rice fast works equally well (where boiled, brown rice is eaten in small bowlfuls whenever required, supplemented with mineral water or home-made potassium broth) but most people prefer the juice fast.

I must emphasise that such fasts must be done under the close supervision of a medical herbalist or naturopath, as they are not suitable for everyone, and you will need an individual examination to determine this.

REGULATING YOUR BLOOD PRESSURE

A simple way to regulate either high or low blood pressure is to take a teaspoonful of cayenne pepper in a glass of warm water three times a day. Build up to this dosage gradually because initially it tastes pretty fiery. Include lots of garlic, buckwheat (for its rutin content), sprouted alfalfa and raw foods in the diet and entirely cut out salt, tea, coffee, chocolate, cocoa, alcohol and all strong spices and flavourings except cayenne and garlic. Meals should be small and often and weight needs to be controlled. Exercise is of paramount importance. This should be done under supervision if obesity is a problem. Aim for a minimum of forty minutes three or four times a week. Avoid hot showers and baths and use instead warm showers alternated with cold showers of two minutes each, repeating several times and finishing with a cold shower.

Lecithin will help emulsify fat in the bloodstream and is available in granules from health food shops. Garlic has the same effect. Always remember that high blood pressure can be triggered by emotions and so stress, fear and prolonged nervous tension need to be taken into consideration and reduced, where possible.

High Blood Pressure Tonic

The formation I use to regulate high blood pressure gradually, strengthen the heart, protect the arteries and improve the circulation is:

Six parts: *One part:*
hawthorn berries   *dandelion*
Three parts: *rosemary*
motherwort   *hyssop*
          nettles

I make this up as a tincture and generally prescribe sixty drops three times a day. If further help for the kidneys is needed, I may also prescribe the kidney detox routine (see page 64–5).

A vegan diet to remove plaquing from the arteries is also a sensible precaution.

• ANGINA •

Coronary heart disease will usually show itself as angina (that is chest pain, especially on exertion). I have already talked about the role of diet in promoting heart disease. A diet high in saturated fats coupled with smoking are the major factors associated with any kind of heart disease. The quickest way to heal those clogged arteries is to embark upon a strict vegan diet coupled with monitored graded exercise, counselling as appropriate and relaxation techniques. I have been able to help patients reduce angina to almost nothing in less than a month using these methods. The exercise does not have to be, and indeed should not be, anything fancy. Begin simply by walking, starting with a few minutes with frequent rests on the flat and gently build up until you are walking at a sustained pace for an hour daily. The cumulative affect on the heart's actions will soon be noticeable. It was George MacAulay Trevelyan, a nineteenth-century doctor who observed, 'I have two doctors, my left leg and my right'. Don't be frightened to use them.

TREATMENT

In treating angina I have put patients on a supervised one-month apple juice fast with garlic and ginger added and plenty of potassium broth, but please don't attempt this yourself without supervision. Remember, vitamin C reduces platelet stickiness in people with coronary heart disease – upwards of 500 mg needs to be taken. Evening primrose oil or borage oil, garlic and ginger, will all help to combat platelet stickiness.

Heart Tonic

An excellent heart tonic which restores and nourishes the heart muscle and circulatory system, dilates the coronary arteries, so increasing blood flow and oxygen to the heart muscle itself and helping with valvular problems, disturbances to the heart's rhythms, palpitations and angina is:

Six parts: *One part:*
hawthorn flower, leaf and berry   *ginger root*
Three parts: *cayenne pepper*
motherwort   *garlic*

I usually prescribe this at between thirty and sixty drops three times a day in tincture form.

• MIGRAINE •

Migraine is one step on from a headache because it involves recurrent headaches with visual and/or gastro-intestinal disturbances so there may be nausea, vomiting and an inability to look at light. Attacks can be preceded by flashes of light, the result of intercerebral vasoconstriction followed by severe head pain confined to one side of the head or eye due to dilation of extracerebral cranial arteries. It is important to get a correct diagnosis before proceeding with treatment since a migraine is much more deep-seated than a headache and will take longer to heal. I have found iridology particularly useful for ascertaining whether there is any liver congestion, intestinal toxaemia or hypoglycaemia, all of which can be the underlying cause of migraine. If I can catch a migraine early enough, I use lobelia in emetic doses because the induction of vomiting will often help to abort a severe migraine. However, this herb is only available on prescription from medical herbalists.

Many studies have shown that certain foods exacerbate migraines including caffeine, sugar, yeast extracts, liver, sausages, broad beans, cheese, pickled herrings, sauerkraut, oranges, bananas, wheat, milk, chocolate and food additives. Smoking, alcohol and the contraceptive pill have also been known to play their part.

Cranial osteopathy and osteopathy may be indicated if muscular spasm or arthritis is present.

HERBAL HELP

If liver congestion is indicated, as I find very often it is, a three-day fast coupled with liver detoxification, castor oil packs and liver cleansing herbs are indicated. Intestinal toxaemia calls for fasting and enemas and in this instance I find chicory root enemas particularly helpful. They can also be used in the early stages of a migraine and sometimes may stop it dead in its tracks. Other herbs which help include violet, peppermint, lavender, feverfew, rosemary, valerian root, vervain, dandelion, motherwort, centaury, ginger root and skullcap. Ginger root is particularly interesting because it is taken as an antiplatelet aggregatory and it seems the blood platelets of migraine sufferers spontaneously come together more than normal between attacks. So ginger tea taken on a regular basis may prove very helpful in these instances.

If you have the kind of migraine which is relieved by a hot water bottle placed on the face or the neck, use herbs which will assist to expand the blood vessels in the head such as peppermint, lavender, rosemary or feverfew. However if you have the kind of migraine that is relieved by ice-packs use valerian, skullcap or motherwort. Infuse or decoct as appropriate any of these as teas and drink three cups per day. Bioforce's Migraine complex is extremely helpful. The usual dose is 30 drops, three times daily.

• IRRITABLE BOWEL SYNDROME •

Irritable bowel syndrome (IBS) is a term that really irritates me. I think it is a catch-all phrase used by doctors when they basically don't know what the problem is. Sometimes they will use the term spastic colon or nervous bowel. The condition is characterised by aches or pains, gas, flatulence, distention and general disturbance in the abdomen as well as disruptive bowel habits with diarrhoea or constipation. But every one of these symptoms can result from one or more of a number of causes. Again I find iridology tests very helpful so that I know exactly what it is I am treating.

CAUSES

IBS may be the result of difficulties with certain foods, the biggest offenders being wheat, corn, dairy products, coffee, tea and citrus fruits. It may be the outcome of a

Candida overgrowth. It may be the result of hypochlorhydria (low stomach acid). When food is not sufficiently broken down in the stomach the bowel simply cannot digest it. Treatment will involve digestive herbs for the stomach and natural digestive enzymes to assist the pancreas. Antibiotics are notorious for disturbing the bacteria and other organisms in the gut and can directly cause IBS. Wheat bran can exacerbate the problem if a person is wheat intolerant. Parasites like giardia lamblia or worms can also be the culprit.

Parasites

When I mention parasites most patients throw up their heads in horror, but in fact they are surprisingly common. One in six people in Britain carries giardia lamblia. This is a minute flagulated protozoa that causes severe fatigue and bowel disturbance including IBS. At their worst they can cause severe malabsorption and total wasting away of the gut lining. Systematically they can cause fatigue, lack of energy, muscle weakness, headaches, sore throats, enlarged lymph glands, night sweats and occasionally fevers.

The problem is that diagnosis of giardia lamblia is very difficult and most routine hospital faeces screenings miss giardiasis ninety-eight per cent of the time. A superficial biopsy of rectal mucosa taken with a small cotton bud swab pressed firmly into the mucosal lining will give you much more accurate results but you would be one of the lucky few if you could convince your doctor to do this for you.

If I suspect worms or parasites may be the problem I will automatically treat with herbs. An artemesia compound is excellent for this purpose and this coupled with a diet rich in garlic, pumpkin seeds (which worms hate) and grapefruit seed extract has excellent results.

Leaky gut syndrome

Leaky gut syndrome (increased intestinal permeability) may be treated by organic linseed soaked in water and drunk, two dessertspoonfuls twice a day (see Resources Directory). Leaky gut syndrome can also be treated by Intestinal Corrective formula 3 and by butyric acid.

DIAGNOSIS

Certainly stress may be a significant factor in IBS but the problem is not all in the mind. While psychotherapy, relaxation techniques and counselling may all help I do urge you to seek an accurate diagnosis first. IBS can be mistaken for coeliac disease, diverticulitis, laxative abuse, lactose intolerance, faecal impaction, Crohn's disease, ulcerative colitis, or even metabolic disorders such as diabetes.

If you cannot find an experienced iridologist please ensure that at the very least you have a rectal swab test to determine whether you have parasites (see above), an enzyme-linked immunosorobent assay, a blood serum test for gut fermentation products, a complete blood count, erythrocyte sedimentation rate and a Heidelberg pH gastric analysis. I would miss out the stool analysis test because they are so ineffective unless done by a conscientious and experienced laboratory technician.

• STOMACH AND DUODENAL ULCERS •

Sometimes known as gastric ulcers, these can be caused by a variety of factors including delayed gastric emptying, over-secretion of hydrochloric acid, deranged stomach lining and a wash back of bile from the duodenum. Ulcers are certainly exacerbated by drugs, particularly aspirin, steroids, non-steroid anti-inflammatory drugs (NSAIDs), cigarettes, alcohol, tea, coffee, vinegar, spices and, of course, prolonged stress. Stomach ulcers are almost unknown in primitive societies which means that an unrefined diet must surely play a large part in their prevention. Only men used to suffer from ulcers but unfortunately they are becoming more apparent as one of the penalties hardworking female executives are now paying for their stressful jobs.

The new research into H pylori has unearthed the presence of a bug called helicobacter pylori in the majority of stomach ulcer cases. They have been found in eighty per cent of stomach ulcers and ninety-five to ninety-eight per cent of duodenal ulcers. Research implicating them in causing ulcers is still very new. It has been suggested that the inflammation caused by the bug appears to interfere with the inhibitory mechanism of acid secretion in the stomach causing an over-production of acids. The H pylori bug is associated with a two- to six-fold increase of gastric cancer. In the Western world the infection occurs in about one-quarter of symptom-free adults increasing to about fifty per cent by the time the person reaches their middle years. It is caught from close contact which is one reason why ulcers appear to run in families.

ALLOPATHIC TREATMENT

Enlightened doctors are beginning to treat this bug with a potent cocktail of chemicals including amoxycillin (an antibiotic), metronidazole (an anti protozoal) and bismuth (an anti ulcer preparation). Any of these used singularly is only about thirty per cent effective, but there will be problems with this chemical arsenal; you can expect to suffer with profound and debilitating diarrhoea, nausea, vomiting, drowsiness, headaches, dizziness, vertigo, irritability, depression, insomnia, confusion, hives, fever and cystitis as well as all the side-effects associated with antibiotics and those associated with bismuth, including the possibility of serious ulceration, stomatitis or kidney failure.

HERBAL HELP

I feel that the risks are far too high a price to pay for what is, in essence, rather a scatter gun approach using three very powerful drugs whose interaction is not fully understood. I would suggest instead a paste made from equal parts of goldenseal and slippery elm together with grapefruit seed extract which has a broad range of anti bacterial activity, including H pylori and campylobacter. It is also anti-fungal and anti-parasitic and, most pleasing of all, it is not toxic and so has no side-effects and is available from Nature's Way and Nature's Herbs (see Resources Directory).

Plenty of raw, fresh garlic juiced in the following drinks will underline its action. Raw, freshly pressed cabbage or potato juice is helpful. Juiced separately or in equal proportions and mixed together the final result is rather unpalatable so mix with celery or carrot juice in proportions of half and half. Aim to drink four or five glasses daily and adhere closely to the food-combining rules as well as a vegan diet. I have helped patients to heal gastric ulcers within four to five weeks if all these instructions are carefully followed. The following powdered herbs mixed singly or proportionately into vegetable juice also help: comfrey, licorice, peppermint, marshmallow, slippery elm.

Dr Christopher, one of the most famous herbalists in America, had great success using cayenne pepper to heal stomach ulcers. He prescribed one heaped teaspoonful three times a day in water.

• DRUG ADDICTION •

More people are addicted to their prescribed drugs than so-called 'addicts' who buy from pushers in the street. All drugs are toxic to some degree and no drug can be pinpointed to affect only the organ it is designed to treat. Some have broad effects and some literally affect every organ in the body. Some of the side-effects are minor nuisances but others can be severely damaging or even fatal. Herbs are useful tools in healing the ravages of drug abuse. Since drug abuse is such a complex social, medical and psychological problem there are no easy answers or simple solutions. Over the years I have observed that a person whose body is filled with artificial substances needs more potent herbs to overcome the resulting tolerance than a person whose body is in a more natural state and, therefore, much more sensitive to the effect of the herb.

My first step is to detoxify the body of all harmful substances including foods such as salt, sugar, caffeine and alcohol. This is a process that has to be done extremely thoroughly but very carefully. Acupuncture is also a wonderful partner in this process.

DETOXIFICATION

As far as street drugs are concerned addicts, by and large, are motivated by the fear of getting sick. Once the addict has made up her mind to change and the motivation to clean up has been established then a world of possibilities is opened up for her in the process of transformation. It is important to explain that the symptoms of detoxification are simply accurate reflections of the healing process. For example, both heroin and methadone depress the respiratory system, so as the drugs are being withdrawn it is not uncommon for an addict to have colds, sniffles, a runny nose etc. Symptoms of general toxicity, such as irritability and depression, also occur as the body throws off toxic substances.

Detox Tea for Drug Addiction

A good detoxification tea is as follows:

Eight parts:	*orange peel*
comfrey leaf	*mullein*
spearmint	*goldenseal*
rosehip	

These herbs should be mixed together and brought to boiling point, but not actually be allowed to boil. Drink six to eight cups a day.

Apart from acupuncture I have also found that supervised short fasts in a relaxing and supportive environment, together with liver and kidney detoxification, counselling and aromatherapy, also helpful. In between the fasts the diet should be kept wholesome. Some addicts respond well to hatha yoga and meditation. I have found yoga very helpful in promoting relaxation for addicts moving away from pills who have difficulty sleeping.

WITHDRAWAL SYMPTOMS

The withdrawal symptoms experienced coming off prescriptive drugs can be just as severe as those coming off heroin, cocaine and methadone, depending on the drug and the length of time the person has been on it. Therefore, all drug withdrawal needs professional supervision. There are certain drugs that cannot be withdrawn (albeit a very small proportion) including cardiac agents used, in particular, for arrhythmias (disturbances to the heart's rhythms), and replacement hormones in endocrine deficiency such as hypothyroidism, diabetes insipidus, diabetes mellitus and an inadequate adrenal cortex. If these drugs are stopped the patient will die and, while alternative treatment is possible, it must be carried out while a doctor regularly monitors the patient.

• ALCOHOL, TOBACCO AND MARIJUANA •

Our two legal drugs, alcohol and tobacco, kill thousands of times more people than illegal street drugs. For every one person who dies from the effects of an illegal drug, thirty die from the effect of alcohol and 400 from tobacco. For every person who dies from smoking, the British government spends £35 on anti-smoking campaigns. For those who die from drinking, the government spends £344 on anti-drinking campaigns, but for every person who dies from illegal street drug use the government spends £1.7 million on anti-drug campaigns.

Legal drugs are undoubtedly much more of a problem than illegal ones. Research shows that a decade ago there were little over 5,000 notified drug addicts in the UK while over 25 million prescriptions were issued for benzodiazepines (see page 208). In the USA one billion prescriptions were issued.

MARIJUANA

Having got the size of the problem into proportion let me tell you that more damage is done to the lungs of marijuana smokers than to heavy tobacco smokers. Its long-term effects can result in constant fatigue and an inability to study, poor memory retention, constant and recurrent small illnesses particularly genital herpes, cold sores on the mouth, skin problems and lack of muscular co-ordination.

My worry with marijuana is that the canabinoid substances in it suppress the immune system and strongly interfere with vital cellular processes. It is psycho-logically as well as physically addictive because the characteristic smell of cannabis smoke is enough to produce the same effect in a habitual marijuana smoker even when all the known active constituents have been removed. Research has also shown that cannabis substances strongly interfere with the synthesis of DNA, RNA and protein. The logical progression of this suggests that more and more children of children of marijuana smokers will be born with genetic defects.

TOBACCO SMOKING

Consider some facts about smoking.

- Cigarettes reduce blood flow, particularly to the hands and feet. It takes six whole hours after the last cigarette to get the blood flow back on an even keel. So if lighting up is the first thing you do when you get out of bed and the last thing you do before sleeping your circulation is probably only normal for about two hours a day.
- Smoking depresses the immune system and this process takes three months to reverse once you have given it up.
- Oseteoporosis has been proven to be aggravated by smoking.
- Menopausal problems are made worse by smoking.
- Smoking inhibits the pancreas and may lead to hypoglycaemia.
- Smoking forces the heart to accelerate to 20–25 beats per minute after only one cigarette, so more oxygen is needed but the poisonous carbon monixide from cigarettes actually forces the oxygen out of the bloodstream. As the result of a reduced supply of oxygen in the bloodstream injuries in smokers heal more slowly that in non-smokers.
- Statistics show that **death from lung cancer in women will overtake death from breast cancer by the year 2,000.**

I am well aware that the majority of smokers are desperate to break their addictive habit and also that smoking has been shown to be more addictive than heroin and cocaine.

LIFE EXPECTANCY

If you need an incentive to spur you on, sit down and work out when you expect to die. Alter the years into months and by doing so your remaining life span will sound shorter. Now we know that each cigarette is estimated to take away eight minutes of life so this means that someone who smokes 20 a day will add one month of life for every year they give up cigarettes. If you smoke 40 a day, this adds up to 16 years less of life. If you don't give up, the quality of life left to you will be severely diminished. Cigarettes contain over 4,000 known toxic poisons, any one of which can kill if taken in sufficient quantity.

GIVING UP SMOKING

Only three per cent of smokers are able to stop smoking on their own. So you might as well relax and recognise the fact that you will almost certainly need professional help and guidance as well as high motivation which only you can supply. Sign up with any programme that has been recommended to you as effective for giving up smoking. Check that it uses the combination of aversion therapy and behaviour modification.

In the initial stages of giving up smoking a prolonged fast, professionally supervised, from seven to 21 days certainly helps to overcome nicotine craving and detoxifies the body rapidly. This is probably best done in a residential naturopathic clinic or a health farm. Any form of hydrotherapy which makes you sweat will help you get rid of nicotine through the skin. Colonics are helpful twice a week for several weeks. Lobelia which contains lobeline and can be prescribed by a medical herbalist has a very similar action to nicotine but is non-addictive. The general dose is 15 drops six times a day but you may take more every time a cigarette is desired. Taken in excess lobelia will cause nausea and may act as an emetic and cause vomiting. This is no bad thing because not only will it clear the stomach of poisons but it will act as an aversion therapy associated with cigarettes.

PASSIVE SMOKING

Passive smoking greatly increases the risk of lung cancer as well as heart disease, nasal sinus cancer and brain tumour. If you are unfortunate enough to work an eight-hour day in the same room as someone who smokes 30 cigarettes a day, you will have passively inhaled five cigarettes and this is enough, in the case of a pregnant woman, to affect the foetus.

ALCOHOLISM

Most of us already know about the long-term effects of too much alcohol including liver disease, high blood pressure, irritability, tremors, slurred speech, the inability to think, depression and fatigue, but few are aware of the adverse effects alcohol has, both on the body's metabolism and on its nutritional state. Obesity is common (a pint of beer is 250 calories) as is damage to the oesophagus, stomach and pancreas. There is an increased risk of gout and increased cholesterol level. Alcoholism can also exacerbate diabetes, heart disease and can damage the brain and nervous system as well as increase the risk of developing cancer of the liver, oesophagus, larynx and mouth.

Women who drink in the weeks before and during pregnancy greatly increase the chances of giving birth to a child with facial deformities or mental retardation.

Some people are allergic to alcohol because of the additives in it or because they have a food intolerance to grape, grain, sugar or yeast. Alcohol is an increasingly common factor in the failure to absorb specific nutrients. The facts speak for themselves. Ninety-five per cent of alcoholics are hypoglycaemic, unsurprising when you consider that alcohol gives an even quicker sugar boost than sucrose. Interestingly, alcohol addiction is extremely rare on a really good wholefood diet.

HERBAL HELP AND TREATMENT

My first line of treatment would be to persuade the patient to take a wholefood diet as well as to prescribe one cup of angelica tea, using both the roots and leaves as a decoction, three times a day. This helps to create a distaste for the taste of alcohol. Evening primrose oil or borage oil (500 mg eight times a day) softens the effects of alcohol withdrawal and as alcohol damages the liver, liver detoxification is called for and kidney detoxification is a desirable adjunct (see pages 63–5).

A wholefood diet should be one eaten little and often and because of the tendency to hypoglycaemia no fruit juice should be taken and all fruit should be eaten with a little protein (for example from seeds, nuts, nut buffers, anything that combines soya and some superfoods, including Spirulina, chlorella and nutritional yeast). The malnutrition that inevitably accompanies alcohol requires heavy supplementation. Use all the superfoods outlined on pp.25–32.

I would urge all alcoholics to join Alcoholics Anonymous; Al-Anon offers support for close friends and family of alcoholics. Al-Alteen works in the same way for the teenage children of alcoholics.

An alcoholic should not be allowed even a teaspoonful of alcohol as it only restimulates the craving, therefore it is wise to check all herbal medication. Alcoholics should not, for example, take herbal tinctures. Check allopathic medication because many cough mixtures are also alcohol based.

• DELIRIUM TREMENS (DTS) •

People often think of the DTs as a joke but it is extremely serious and requires immediate help. It is the result of coming off a high intake of alcohol abruptly. Withdrawal symptoms include mental confusion, memory loss, hallucinations, shaking, sweating, insomnia, agitation, fast pulse and high blood pressure, all of which may go on for as many as four days.

Give one-quarter of a cup of equal parts of skullcap and lady's slipper brewed as a decoction every half hour until the DTs subside. Sweeten it with honey to assist blood sugar levels temporarily. Seek immediate medical attention.

• LIVING IN THE FAST LANE
AND HOW TO GET OUT OF IT •

I love speed and height; roller coaster rides, fast cars, tandem parachuting, and gliding, I have done them all. But my way of thrill seeking and pushing the outer edge of the envelope is temporary and I do ensure that my highs are interspersed with long periods of quiet time spent at a much lower key holidaying and resting. The price many working women are paying for success is very expensive: various addictions, broken marriages, estranged children, ulcers, heart attacks, high blood pressure and even cancer. What you need to ask yourself is do you really want to wake up aged 65 with a gold carriage clock in a big empty house in the suburbs with a husband and children who couldn't care less? The stress in the lives of isolated mothers and working women has a lot to answer for.

I feel the linchpin to getting out of the fast lane and maintaining some sanity is one of a woman's strongest assets, her identification with her family and friends. Of course, work and families are not mutually exclusive. They may be for a short time but not for a whole life. The only way women who love their jobs and have a family are going to survive the stress of two jobs is to ensure that their partners pitch in and that they have plenty of help with the housework. Men's greater experience in the business world has always given them the greater ability to integrate their personal and professional lives but women are getting there with women's networks.

QUALITY TIME

You have probably heard it many times before but it is worth repeating. It is essential that you make time for yourself. If you have a partner make sure that you set time aside just for you. This is particularly important if you are a mother. To stay alive and healthy a sexual relationship must be guarded carefully against the assaults of offspring and outside interests. Weekends and holidays for two, even farming the children out for a night every now and then, are essential. Studies show that the potential axis of the family, the husband–wife relationship, is bent or broken by the presence of children and that this is both a description and a cause of marital dissatisfaction.

It may be that the division is inevitable. That is the cost of having children and raising them; the price satisfaction may bring. If this were so most of us would go on having children anyway, presumably swapping one kind of satisfaction for another and enriching our lives by the differing qualities of the two experiences of parenthood and marriage. But it is possible that this division is not necessary, that children demand it of us, or women prefer it, or even that current childcare theory advocates it, or men allow it, or because we accord the marriage relationship no conscious priorities. It is very easy when there are children to let a marriage become expendable. It can so easily slip away without us fighting for it. While everyone has heard a great deal about neglected children it is certainly equally true that there are a great many neglected marriages. Studies show that couples are happiest with each other before the children are born and after the children have left the nest.

If I had to review one of the greatest assets of my life it is my friends. Friendships, well handled, will see you through the bad times and help you rejoice through the good times. Set time aside for them.

ADRENAL MAINTENANCE

I am well aware that all of this sage advice may not be possible to follow because we don't live in a perfect world. Prolonged stress not only batters our nervous systems, it can also do insidious damage to our glandular system, particularly to our adrenal glands. However, two possible benefits derive from the stable functioning of adrenal hormones. Firstly, abundant energy and secondly, a super-charged immune system able to fight off disease quickly, completely, and with the minimum of fuss. If you simply cannot be bothered about anything and life is just too short even to try, it means that your adrenalin is low. The danger here is not only to your personality but to your ability to fight off disease attacks quickly and completely. People will often say to me, 'I wish I had your energy to do all the things you do', and my question is, 'So, what is stopping you? Fear? Hopelessness? Despair? Laziness? Lack of self-esteem? Alcohol? Drugs? Smoking?' There is no one natural remedy for restoring sexual drive. Certainly good nutrition helps, particularly magnesium and zinc, but an abundance of adrenal hormone will always stimulate the ovaries into action. Women have better vaginal lubrication when they are adrenally well stocked.

Adrenal Tonic

The following formulation is designed to restore hormonal function, support the adrenal glands, regulate blood sugar and increase the body's resistance to disease, so helping counteract stress. It is also rather good for jet lag if taken a week before the flight and a week after.

Two parts: *wild oats*
Siberian ginseng root   *bladderwrack*
One part: *gotu kola*
echinacea

This should be made as a tincture. The dosage I would give an adult normally is fifteen drops three times a day.

Formula for Chronic Exhaustion

The following formulation will help the adrenal glands by nourishing and supporting them in the long term. This is useful when stress has been chronic.

One part: *Half a part:*
ginger   *damiana*
cayenne pepper   *lavender*
dandelion   *St John's Wort.*
milk thistle

Take Three size 0 capsules morning and evening.

Alternatively, try the Ginkgo Biloba marketed by Nature's Plus (see Resources Directory).

• CANDIDIASIS •

Candida Albicans is a yeast that lives in the digestive tract of everyone. It is only when our immune system has become compromised by antibiotics, steroids, poor diet or prolonged stress, environmental chemicals or a continual damp climate that the form of the yeast changes to a fungal one. When this happens long threads, called hyphae, start growing and attack the wall of the intestine making it permeable to some of the larger protein molecules that normally cannot penetrate it (like those found in wheat and dairy products) and these are then passed into the bloodstream causing an allergic reaction.

SYMPTOMS

The symptoms of an overgrowth of Candida albicans read like a hypochondriac's dream or an alternative therapist's nightmare, depending on which way you look at it. But the sadness of it is that, in my experience, candida is frighteningly common. Indeed I believe it may infect, one way or another, almost a quarter of my patients. Symptoms include:

- infections of the skin, showing redness, itching and swelling;
- nails, which become hardened, thickened, grooved and often brownish coloured;
- vaginal infections characterised by itching, redness and white discharge;
- muscle weakness, painful or swollen joints and poor co-ordination;
- mood swings, depression, lethargy, de-personalisation (a sense of spaciness) and, unsurprisingly, a loss of interest in sex, as well as anxiety and irritability;
- feeling tired or drowsy.

- a variety of food intolerances and uncomfortable reactions to things like perfumes or certain chemical smells;
- bloating, heartburn, constipation, bad breath;
- chest pains, shortness of breath, dizziness, easy bruising;
- frequent headaches which manifest themselves as pressure above or behind the eyes or ears;
- cystitis which in spite of swabs shows up as negative;
- PMS or erratic periods.

Now you can understand why I say that having ploughed your way through that little list you **must** seek accurate diagnosis. In my experience iridology is not accurate but Vega testing (depending on the experience of the operator) is. Biolab have also developed a gut fermentation test and refined it to a degree where they can distinguish yeast from a bacterial overgrowth. They will only accept references from doctors (see Resources Directory).

To give a rough guideline, if you look at that entire list and can circle seven or eight symptoms you should get yourself accurately diagnosed.

TREATMENT AND HERBAL HELP

My treatment begins with a good wholefood vegan diet, including at least fifty per cent raw foods. Practitioners who preclude yeast, as so many do, puzzle me. The difference between food yeast and the candida organism is rather like the difference between a bay tree and a monkey puzzle tree. While I might advocate the exclusion of brewer's yeast and substitute an inactive nutritional yeast, I certainly do not exclude fruits and vegetables from the diet. I do ask patients to take plenty of organic olive oil and eat plenty of garlic. I have found a very good way of eating garlic in huge quantities is to slice up the raw cloves and eat them piece by piece with mouthfuls of ripe fresh pears. Another method is to liquidise the garlic with a cupful of organic apple juice and one inch of peeled fresh ginger. This actually makes a very pleasant drink.

Sealing a permeable gut can also be done successfully with Intestinal Corrective Formula 3 (see page 73). Paracidin can be useful if the yeast spores have escaped into the respiratory tract or the sinuses. I do insist that the patients avoid alcohol, tea, coffee and cocoa, all of which suppress the proper working of the immune system. I insist that all fruit be fresh and eaten whole, as fruit juice is too concentrated in sugar and that any sweeteners like honey, maple syrup and molasses, as well as sugar, are entirely omitted from the diet.

Apart from garlic there is a wide range of herbs that are extremely effective against fungus including black walnut, T-tree, horsetail. Support of the immune system (after all one of the precursors of Candida albicans is a prolonged siege of the immune system) includes echinacea, Pau D'arco, and various medicinal mushrooms.

Being a trained colonic therapist as well as a medical herbalist, I have used colonic therapy with great success with Candida albicans, providing the gut has not proved leaky, and hydrotherapy, particularly pyrotechnic treatments, have proved invaluable for stimulating an exhausted immune system.

• POST-VIRAL FATIGUE SYNDROME •

If you haven't heard of this you will have almost certainly heard of ME (myalgic encephalomyeltis), chronic mononucleosis, Epstein-Barr virus syndrome, all of which add up to extreme debilitation for the unfortunate patient and a huge amount of controversy among doctors. My feeling about this syndrome is dichotomous. After ensuring an accurate diagnosis has been made I have been fortunate enough to inspire hundreds of patients into following all the right instructions to heal themselves. On the other hand so many people suffering from this chronic debility have run the gauntlet with the medical profession and been dismissed as hypochondriacs, that by the time they reach me they are in a state of profound spiritual and mental depression which makes them very difficult to counsel.

CAUSE

Post viral fatigue syndrome, as the name suggests, is the result of a malfunctioning immune system which has been hit with one or several consecutive viruses and consequently has never been able to recover. Unsurprisingly, very many people who get viral fatigue find it coupled to a Candida albicans overgrowth. A cardiologist at London's Charing Cross Hospital, far from concurring with this theory, feels that it is simply a result of chronic exhaustion. My feeling is that he may well be right because all of the patients I have worked with, who have this syndrome, have been high-achieving go-getters working very long hours. This alone is enough to make an over-stressed immune system eventually start protesting.

The latest research now points to the fact that ME is probably the result of a persistent viral infection resulting in an overactive immune system. Sleep disorders are now believed to be important in the cause of the syndrome and there is some suggestion that ME and polio might be linked. Post-polio syndrome consists of progressive muscular weakness and fatigue and persistent viruses all occurring some twenty-five or even thirty years after recovery from paralytic polio. Couple all these factors with others that may act as triggers, like bacterial infections, injury, hormonal changes and psychological stress, and you have a picture which may include inflammation throughout the central nervous system, disturbances in blood flow to the brain (brain scans of some patients show the same abnormality shown in scans of AIDS patients), noticeable hormonal and nervous system changes, all manifesting as muscle pain aggravated by very limited movement, nausea and flu-like feelings, as well as depression. ME can also be linked to malabsorption; B12, B6, chromium, zinc and magnesium deficiencies are common. Herbs for the pancreas as well as digestive enzymes can often help in these instances, encouraging better absorption.

Giardia also needs to be tested (see page 165) as I have found parasitic infection surprisingly common in my post-viral fatigue syndrome patients.

All these factors have to be taken into account but I have had great success with co-operative patients following hydrotherapy regimes, dietary alterations, especially those which include a lot of freshly squeezed organic carrot juice, skin brushing twice daily, attention to the bowel with the various bowel herbs (see pages 71–74), help with candida and giardia if it was indicated, lots of superfoods listed on pages 25–32 and echinacea given in high quantities, together with devil's claw and evening primrose oil or borage seed oil. Initially I often give, depending on the weight of the patient, 350 drops of echinacea a day, spread out over the course of a day, together with ten to fifteen drops of devil's claw three times a day, and a minimum of 1,500 mg of evening primrose oil before bed. I give brief rests for a few days at the end of every fortnight from the echinacea.

Devil's claw, Harpagophytum procumbens, is used for its anti-inflammatory properties as well as for its specific indication for myalgia and its extraordinary ability to alter the metabolic process in the body.

• DENTAL AMALGAMS •

Research has shown that the mercury commonly used in fillings is toxic. More than 12,000 papers on the dangers of amalgam have been published but so far the results have failed to alter the opinions of the majority of the dental profession. Let me give you the following facts.

- Mercury is associated with sclerotic diseases including multiple sclerosis.
- There is growing evidence that mercury rather than aluminium is the largest trace element found in the brains of victims of Alzheimer's disease.
- There seems to be an association between a high resistance to antibiotics and high mercury content. This is interesting because research into problems with very severe candida suggest that the yeast reacts to the mercury in amalgam fillings creating methyl mercury in the digestive tract, which is far more toxic than ordinary mercury, and so conjuring a situation where candida is much tougher to eradicate.
- The removal of root canal fillings which were done with amalgam have been shown to improve kidney and heart disease in the majority of patients suffering from these. However, not all people react unfavourably to such root canal fillings; much depends on heredity.
- Mercury lowers T-lymphocyte cells.
- Mercury fillings in pregnant women have been found to affect the foetus and the filling of teeth of pregnant women in Sweden with mercury has now been totally banned.

In all the years I have been in practice I have accumulated a lot of practical experience as to the dangers of mercury. Before I give you some examples let me emphasise that by no means does everyone react badly to mercury fillings and these should be tested by someone qualified and experienced in this field. I cannot emphasise enough how important it is to get the fillings removed in the right sequence. Both Levenson and Huggins, the leaders in this field, insist that the most negatively charged fillings be taken out first. In addition to this a very strict protocol must be followed so do go to a dentist who is recommended by Jack Levenson in this field. Any dentist will not do. In fact, those who rush off to dentists to have their amalgam fillings replaced willy nilly often get sicker because the protocol has not been observed and they suffer from an onslaught of mercury vapours.

Other recommendations include the use of a rubber dam together with high volume extraction and high speed cutting with a water coolant spray while the patient has her eyes covered with damp cotton wool or wrap-around goggles and a nose piece supplying oxygen.

If the patient has been diagnosed as being extremely highly sensitive to mercury (and tests done in advance can ascertain this) they should be treated with six grams ascorbate vitamin C mixed into water at the first signs of any adverse reaction. I always start my own patients on very high oral nutritional therapy including extremely high doses of spirulina and Intestinal Corrective Formula 3 and the following heavy metal detoxification treatment. Working in conjunction with Philip Wander in Manchester, England I have observed some really excellent results with this programme coupled with his good and experienced dentistry.

Heavy Metal Detoxifying Programme

1. Six teaspoonfuls of Intestinal Corrective Formula 3, or pectin available in cooked apples. Eat 1lb (0.45 Kg) of the cooked puree daily. Alternatively, take six teaspoonfuls of pectin powder in juice daily.

2. Take three charcoal tablets three times a day with meals.

3. Take one cup of sprouted seeds daily or two tablespoonfuls of Superfood stirred into juice morning and evening (see Resources Directory).

4. Six cloves of raw garlic a day (see tip on p. 174 to take that amount comfortably).

5. Two tablespoonfuls of lecithin granules a day.

6. One cup of the following decoction with each meal:

Three parts:	*yellow dock*
burdock root	*One/two parts:*
gypsy weed	*plantain*

This routine should be followed for at least a week before the dental work begins and for six weeks afterwards. Alternatively use Pronatura's Dentox (see Resources Directory). This programme is also excellent for detoxifying the body of lead, cadmium and aluminium.

CHAPTER 12:

HOLISTIC HERBAL FIRST AID

———

Every responsible household should have a well-stocked first-aid cabinet at home, as well as a first-aid travel bag at the ready in case of an emergency. This chapter is not designed to qualify anyone in first aid, nor does it contain detailed instructions for bandaging, splinting, suturing or setting broken bones. All these useful skills can be learned at a first-aid class, so enroll at least one member of the family. Your local branch of the Red Cross runs these regularly. Most people are terrified at the thought of an accident occurring and wouldn't know how to cope if one did. By learning the most effective way to respond to any accident you can be relieved of this terror, and attendance at a first-aid course is the first step to doing this.

• VITAL FIRST AID •

There are two accident situations when speedy action is vital: when a person has stopped breathing due to choking, electric shock or drowning, or when a person is bleeding severely due to a large cut or puncture wound.

BREATHING

If breathing has stopped, resuscitation should begin within minutes. This type of resuscitation is taught at every first-aid class.

BLEEDING

If someone is bleeding severely, ensure there is no foreign body in the wound and then apply firm pressure. Raise and support injured limb. Only very serious bleeding from a major artery requires the use of a tourniquet, which should preferably be applied by someone properly trained in first aid. Improper use of a tourniquet can result in blood vessel and nerve damage.

• BASIC ITEMS FOR YOUR FIRST-AID CABINET •

Ensure that your first-aid kit contains scissors, a thermometer, safety pins, tweezers, cotton balls, sterile eye pads, crepe bandages, absorbent dressing, sterile gauze dressings, a small pack of paper tissues, perforated bandages, stretchy bandages and outterfly bandages.

● LIST OF ESSENTIAL HERBAL PREPARATIONS FOR A FIRST-AID CABINET ●

Ensure you have a small supply of each of the following herbs in their dried and powdered form:
  cayenne pepper
  chaparral
  false unicorn
  slippery elm
  comfrey
  charcoal (in powder or tablet form)
  intestinal corrective no 3
  intestinal corrective no 1 or 2 (capsule form decanted and clearly labelled in a
    self-sealed plastic bag)

Include the following tinctures:
  arnica
  cayenne pepper
  echinacea
  goldenseal
  plantain
  ginger
  nervine
  digestive

Include the following essential oils:
  lavender
  rosemary
  T-tree
  St John's wort
  clove

Ensure you have a bottle of Bach Flower Rescue Remedy, Rescue Remedy cream, comfrey ointment and marigold cream, also a small bottle of syrup of ipecacuana, some vitamin E oil in capsule form, a small jar of organic runny honey, a bulb of fresh garlic, a bottle of witch hazel, a bottle of Composition Essence, some Olbas oil, the tincture for insomnia (see page 191), and a tincture for indigestion (see page 188). Put any oils and tinctures in 1 fl (30 ml) brown glass bottles with small droppers.

• CONDITIONS SUITABLE FOR FIRST AID •

This section of the book will help you to deal with the most commonly occurring conditions as far as first aid is concerned and offers advice on what to do until a doctor can be reached. Most accidents are not serious and there are rarely true emergencies in the sense that it is important to act or get help immediately. In nearly every accident, in my experience, you have enough time to comfort the victim and calm them down, as well as calming yourself down of course, before you begin to evaluate the extent of the injury. **Calming down is the first important step in treating most accidents, so take some Rescue Remedy yourself before offering any help.**

BLEEDING

Haemorrhage

To stop haemorrhaging internally, mix one teaspoonful of cayenne pepper in a quarter of a glass of warm water and drink it. As a vaginal douche, mix one ounce (30 grams) to one pint (600 ml) of warm water and administer it lukewarm and unstrained. Externally, apply the powder direct to the wound. It is rich in vitamin A and so acts as an excellent disinfectant but do check that the wound is clean first.

Nosebleed

For a nosebleed, sniff dry cayenne.

Stomach bleeding

Stomach bleeding may be soothed by slippery elm gruel. Make this as an infusion but initially mix the powder with only a little hot water to make a paste, adding hot water slowly, and stirring vigorously to prevent unappetising lumps from forming. Then eat the gruel.

BURNS

First-degree burns

For first-degree burns (burns that affect the outer skin only causing redness, dryness, blistering and mild swelling) immerse the burn **immediately** in cold running water or rub it with ice-cubes until all the pain has gone. This rapid response will stop blisters from forming and will modify any tissue damage. If the burn is extremely mild, cut a juicy leaf off an aloe vera plant, open it and apply the jelly-like contents directly to the burn. Alternatively, soak a piece of gauze in aloe vera juice and wrap it around the burn. Lavender oil, comfrey ointment, St John's wort oil, marigold cream or the contents of vitamin E oil capsules are also helpful, but see p. 53 for contra-indications with St John's wort oil.

Second-degree burns

For second-degree burns which involve the lower skin layers and may produce mottling, blisters or swelling, follow the same initial hydrotherapy as for first-degree burns, then spread the vitamin E oil over the burn (use several capsules if the area is large). This will protect the skin while you prepare a paste of equal parts of powdered comfrey, runny organic honey and vitamin E oil. Spread this evenly over the burn and **leave it on**. Cover it with gauze and a bandage. Do not attempt to peel it off. Add more paste as the skin absorbs it. Continue to do this for a few days until all pain and swelling has subsided. If for any reason you do have to remove it (and try to avoid this) soak it off with a warm decoction of goldenseal. Keep the burn out of the sun. As soon as the skin is strong enough, skin brush daily (see p. 61). Meanwhile, drink plenty of carrot juice to accelerate the healing of the burn.

Acid burns

For acid burns flush the area immediately with one pint (600 ml) of cold water in which you have stirred one teaspoonful of bicarbonate of soda. Apply poultices of ice-cold witch-hazel, preferably non-alcoholic, until the pain subsides and then smear with copious amounts of vitamin E oil, replenishing this every hour.

Third-degree burns

Third-degree burns, which involve the full thickness of the skin, require **immediate medical supervision** as these injuries can lead to severe loss of fluids and electrolytes; shock and death are even possible. Powdered comfrey root stirred into any fruit or vegetable juice and taken internally will accelerate the healing. On your way to hospital continue to soak the area in ice-cold water.

Tongue burns

If you burn your tongue sprinkle a few grains of sugar on it, and repeat until the pain subsides.

BRUISES

Apply an ice-cold compress of witch-hazel to the bruise on a piece of gauze liberally sprinkled with tincture of arnica. Ice-packs are also useful. I keep cubes of frozen non-alcoholic witch-hazel in my deep freezer which is an incredibly effective way to use this herb on bruises. Do not put ice directly on to the skin; always wrap it in a clean piece of gauze first.

If you find you are bruising easily you may be short of vitamin C and its complexes, including hesperedin which is present in the white pith of citrus fruit.

CATARRH

Fast for three days on apple juice and potassium broth. Make a salt glow by mixing one pound of fine sea salt in just enough water to make a slurry. Have a warm shower and then, while you are still in the shower, rub the salt firmly all over the body in brisk circular movements. Finish with an ice-cold shower. Then you will find out why this is called a glow!

Eat plenty of raw garlic. Do a facial steam with olbas oil. This can also be burned with a vaporiser at night. Apply alternate hot and cold compresses locally to the troublesome area or use forceful hot and cold showers. If the catarrh is very deep-seated you might consider trying the master cleanser diet for a minimum of ten days. It consists of fasting on a mug of hot water with the juice of a lemon or lime squeezed into it, with two tablespoonfuls of maple syrup and one-quarter of a teaspoonful of cayenne pepper added. Renew and ingest this drink as often as desired during the course of a day and drink plenty of water.

Obviously, you will need to avoid foods that cause excessive catarrh. These include all dairy products and refined carbohydrates as well as any local irritations including fumes, chemicals and allergens.

CHILBLAINS

Unbroken chilblains

Provided the chilblains are not broken, hot mustard foot baths followed by cold dips are very helpful. Use one tablespoonful of mustard powder to a bucket of hot water, so that the soak reaches to the knee. Repeat this hot–cold treatment eight times daily.

Alternatively, mix equal parts of cayenne pepper and corn starch and put this in your socks. A simpler method is snow walking. Walk barefoot on an even stretch of snow for ten seconds, gradually increasing to two or three minutes longer. It is important that you go outside without having warmed yourself up first and that you are well covered except for your feet. Dry your feet by rubbing them well with your hands, not with a towel, and go to bed.

Sprouted buckwheat made into a porridge will assist the circulation by elasticising the arteries.

Nelson's chilblain ointment is excellent if the chilblains are not broken.

Broken chilblains

If chilblains are broken, soak them in a warm infusion of dried marigold flowers then cover them with a poultice of the strained-out petals, securing this in place with a bandage. Leave the poultice on the skin overnight and repeat the procedure until healed. Once the skin is healed, apply marigold ointment until the redness has completely disappeared.

COLD SORES

Apply goldenseal tincture or T-tree oil directly and eat plenty of garlic.

Take equal parts of skullcap and goldenseal in tincture form internally. The normal dose is ten drops hourly until the cold sore has stopped hurting and then ten drops three times daily until it has completely cleared.

COLDS

A cold that is properly managed should last for only two days and should flow purposefully and freely. Think of it as a natural purification process. Any cold that is discouraged and suppressed with chemical remedies may drag on in one form or another for two or three months.

The correct old adage should be 'if you feed a cold, you will have to starve a fever'. So you should fast on fruit juice, potassium broth and herbal teas for two to three days. Do not extend the fasting beyond this time as it tends to prolong the cold. Instead go on to a diet which includes plenty of onions, garlic and citrus fruits.

One of the most effective teas I have found for a cold is ginger tea with honey, lemon, a generous pinch of cayenne pepper and a crushed clove of garlic in each mug.

Use hot mustard foot baths to decongest the head and a salt water douche into the nose using a nasal spray to open up and decongest the sinuses.

Alternatively, facial steam inhalations using Olbas oil or thyme oil are helpful, as is the ready made Composition Essence which consists of elderflowers, peppermint and yarrow. Use two teaspoonfuls in a mug of hot water and sip the mixture hot. Drink frequently.

As the cold is a viral infection, it can be effectively treated by echinacea tincture. Take one teaspoonful of the tincture in a little water every two hours. If the throat is sore, spray this mixture neat down the throat or gargle with it.

COUGHS

I have found tincture of plantain (ten drops in water as needed) and garlic or onion syrup (one tablespoonful as often as needed) both extremely effective for treating coughs. A cough is simply nature's way of clearing an infection in the bronchial tubes where bacteria is being immobilised, so protecting the lungs from damage.

Both coughs and sore throats are often helped by a short fast on apple juice or a diet using warm vegetable broth and soupy grains. To make onion or garlic syrup, cover several finely sliced onions or three to four bulbs of sliced and peeled garlic with organic liquid honey. Low heat at under 130°F for several hours and strain and cool it. Hold the syrup in the mouth and let it trickle slowly down the throat.

You can massage the chest with anti-spasmodic tincture (see page 191), olbas oil diluted with a little olive oil or a ginger compress.

If the cough is prolonged and merely irritating make a decoction of equal parts of wild cherry bark, aniseed and wild lettuce and drink a cup full of this reheated and liberally laced with organic honey every two hours.

Increase your intake of garlic to six or seven cloves a day.

If any cough lasts more than a week please seek further help from a professional medical herbalist, a naturopath or a doctor. It may need further investigation.

CONSTIPATION

See p. 68–9

CRAMPS

To treat muscular cramps, massage in tiger balm or the deep heat treatment (see Resources Directory). Both relax tight muscles amazingly fast.

If the cramp is in the legs take a hot bath and then stand facing a wall with your toes placed twenty-seven inches away, keeping your heels in contact with the floor. Lean into the wall until you can feel a stretch all the way down your calves, hold for ten seconds, release for five seconds, and repeat three times. If you do this two to three times a day faithfully for a month it will also help to alleviate pain in the lower back.

CUTS AND MINOR WOUNDS

If the wound is bleeding copiously place it in ice-cold water or apply cayenne pepper directly. Both will arrest the bleeding and reduce inflammation. Ensure the cut is absolutely clean. Proper cleansing is vital to help the wound heal easily and to prevent infection. Do ensure the wound is not so deep that it needs emergency micro-surgery. You may consider a cut deep enough if it goes through the skin and is long enough so that the sides of the cut separate and do not stay together. When a cut is this deep you will see shiny connective tissue or yellow globules of fat in the wound. If you are in any doubt about this go to your emergency accident unit and have it examined.

Having cleansed the wound properly to ensure rapid healing and prevent infection, apply T-tree or thyme oil neat. All of them sting like crazy but they will stop any infection. A poultice of powdered comfrey mixed with a little honey will accelerate the healing. If the cut is very superficial use comfrey ointment.

If a large flap of skin is cut off, such as a fingertip, pressure should be applied to the cut to stop the bleeding. The piece of skin should then be put into ice-cold water or salt water (half a teaspoonful of salt to two pints (1.2 litres) of water) and taken to the doctor. Generally it is possible to stitch the flap back on. However, on two occasions I have used anti-infective tincture followed by a poultice of wheatgerm oil, powdered comfrey and honey, and healed such wounds without any scarring at all.

If the bleeding is copious and difficult to stop take a quarter of a teaspoonful of cayenne pepper in warm water, internally, and apply a tourniquet externally.

DIARRHOEA

Diarrhoea is caused by a substance irritating the colon so badly that peristalsis goes into overdrive in an attempt to expel it. However, chronic diarrhoea which goes on for several days or recurs persistently needs professional help. **Any diarrhoea in infancy which does not clear up within twenty-four hours needs immediate and urgent medical attention**.

Fast on warm water with whole organic lemons pulped into it and honey. The pectin in the lemons is very useful for neutralising toxins. Drink as much infused blackberry leaf tea as you can because it is very astringent and will help to restore the tone and function of the bowel. It also stops dehydration and the subsequent loss of electrolytes. Eat plenty of raw garlic for its anti-viral antibiotic effect. Alternatively, if the thought of garlic makes you heave, take Bioforce's Tormenta-vena, ten drops hourly in water, until the diarrhoea stops.

Alternatively, liquidise the Intestinal Correction Formula 3 in plenty of apple juice and drink this. A minimal dose should be six teaspoonfuls a day (see p.73). When you begin eating again, try well-ripened bananas mashed into soya yogurt or puréed apple liberally laced with cinnamon.

At the end of an acute episode of diarrhoea, if you haven't been able to rehabilitate the flora (see Resources Directory) of the colon with garlic because you felt too sick to eat it, then take one capsule of bioacidophilus morning and evening.

EARACHE

Ears are very delicate, sensitive and complex organs and can easily be permanently damaged by neglect or inappropriate treatment so if you are in any doubt at all about the cause of an earache please consult your doctor. If the earache is the result of a chill, apply a raw grated onion poultice over the back and sides of the neck, securing it with a cotton bandage.

Put a few drops of mullein oil or garlic oil into both ears, even if the earache is only in one ear, and plug with a cotton ball.

A hot foot bath may help the pain of earache, as will any source of heat locally applied, for instance lying on a hot water bottle that is well-wrapped in a towel.

FIBROSITIS

This is sometimes known as muscular rheumatism and is the result of inflammation of the tendons and of the connective tissues covering the muscles.

If the attack is acute and caused by trauma, use ice compresses leaving them on for forty minutes at a time and repeating every two hours for the first forty-eight hours. Then alternate hot and cold compresses, massaging anti-spasmodic tincture into the affected area first. If there is no swelling, hot Epsom salt compresses can be used. I make a deep tissue repair treatment oil which is excellent for any muscular strains or injuries. It is too complex to be made at home but it contains marigold, arnica, St John's wort, cayenne and ginger.

If the pain is chronic and long established you need to seek the help of a professional; meanwhile massage in tiger balm or deep tissue repair oil and take anti-spasmodic tincture internally, ten drops every half hour, to ease the pain and inflammation.

Vitamin C is known to help protect against connective tissue injuries.

HEADACHES AS THE RESULT OF TENSION

Stress can quickly turn painless muscle tension into a headache. If the stress persists toxins will accumulate in the neck and shoulders and you may suffer with osteoarthritis. Cupping a telephone between the neck and shoulder, which is one of my sins, while writing certainly exacerbates this problem. A few big, slow, half head rolls sitting upright with the shoulders relaxed helps here.

Chronic headaches can also be the result of liver congestion, poor circulation, constipation, hypoglycaemia, food intolerance, sinusitis, arthritis, spinal lesions, anaemia, the side-effects of a lumbar puncture, meningitis, a brain tumour, high blood pressure and eye strain. As you can see some of these are serious so investigate a chronic headache by consulting a doctor before resorting to self-medication with herbs. A severe headache with vomiting, for example, may be the result of intra-cerebral haemorrhage which is an emergency.

If the headache is simply the result of tension, place a steaming hot wet towel round the back of the neck and simultaneously put your feet in a basin full of hot water. Alternatively, take a brisk walk making sure your hands, feet, head and neck are well covered and breathe deeply while you do so. On your return take ten drops of anti-spasmodic tincture (see p.191) every half hour in a cup of hot peppermint or chamomile tea.

HEART ATTACK

In an emergency, while waiting for the ambulance or doctor, administer three teaspoonfuls of cayenne pepper in warm water initially, (this to be drunk all at once) and then half a teaspoonful every fifteen minutes in warm water. If the patient cannot swallow, massage Rescue Remedy into the wrists, tongue and lips. You might want to take some yourself. It is very helpful for allaying shock and fear. I have heard of it being successfully administered in hospital by a doctor through an intravenous drip. If you have time apply a steaming hot towel over the patient's heart for no more than three minutes, while bathing the face briefly with ice-cold water.

HICCUPS

As this tends only to be a problem when food is fermenting in the stomach, the first rule is to adhere meticulously to the rules of food combining (see p. 32).

I'm sure you have heard the cure of drinking cold water out of the wrong side of a glass. Surprisingly, if often works very effectively. If it doesn't, take the digestive tincture directly on the tongue, fifteen drops as needed, or sip a cup of fennel tea. Alternatively, eat a lemon wedge soaked in angostura bitters. Breathing into a paper bag, not a plastic one, often helps.

INDIGESTION, OTHERWISE KNOWN AS HEARTBURN, DYSPEPSIA OR GASTRITIS

Indigestion is a somewhat vague term embracing any kind of abdominal discomfort after eating. To my mind it is one of the easiest complaints to rectify, without even having to resort to herbal medicine, if eating habits are altered and the food combining rules are followed. Meals should always be eaten in a calm, quiet atmosphere at a leisurely pace.

1. Chew properly and thoroughly.
2. Do not take liquid with meals unless it is a medicinal herbal tea or a potassium broth. If soup is being taken as part of the meal leave a fifteen-minute gap before going on to the rest of the meal.
3. Avoid salt and all spices, sugar, tea, coffee, alcohol, soda, refined carbohydrates, including fried foods, and anything else which you suspect acts as a gastric irritant.
4. Do not eat excessively hot or ice-cold foods.
5. Never eat if you are distressed. If you are really hungry, sip a glass of vegetable juice, which should be at room temperature, or a cup of potassium broth until you have completely calmed down.
6. Do not eat if you are ill.
7. Eat in unhurried, relaxed surroundings. No arguments at the table!
8. Eat small meals and always leave the table feeling you have room for just a little more.
9. If food is eaten too soon after a previous meal the natural pace of the digestive process will be disrupted, so allow two hours' respite after a fruit meal, three hours after a vegetable one and if you have completely messed up your food combining do not eat so much as a peanut for five hours. However, plenty of liquids may be taken.
10. If none of this helps, investigate the possibility of an intolerance to dairy products or wheat, or check with a professional to see if you have candidiasis. Distortion of the thoracic vertebrae can affect the stomach and will need to be rectified by an osteopath.

     As an iridologist I find it easy to determine if the stomach is hypo or hyper acid. In my experience most people over forty become deficient in digestive enzymes and these will help an hypo acid stomach (see Resources Directory). For hyper acidity try chewing four slippery elm tablets after meals, or three charcoal tablets, or drink an infusion of meadow sweet tea. If the indigestion is acute the obvious thing to do is not eat any more food and fast on something bland such as carrot juice with a touch of fresh ginger root in it if you are thirsty or hungry. A tea made of equal parts of fennel, peppermint and dill will facilitate digestion after a meal. This is much better for you than coffee which simply overloads and distresses the liver.

I absolutely abhor the use of commercial antacids. Those made of sodium bicarbonate are designed to relieve the excess acid which causes indigestion and heartburn by neutralising the gastric acid in the stomach. However, if used regularly they disrupt the natural acid-alkaline balance of the body, causing alkalosis which can, if exacerbated by a substantial intake of dairy products, result in irreversible kidney damage. Milk can actually increase hydrochloric acid secretion in some people which can make the symptoms far worse. Besides this, many antacids contain aluminium, an excessive intake of which is extremely poisonous. Aluminium accumulates in the liver and interferes with its function. It affects the kidneys causing nephritis and degeneration and may cause non-specific joint problems by affecting bone metabolism. This is because an aluminium overload also affects the central nervous system, particularly the parathyroid. So please, avoid antacids as far as possible.

INSOMNIA

We are only able to heal ourselves when we are asleep, so sleep is vital for rejuvenation. Besides this, our dreams can carry out the nightly task of sifting through the day's unsettled problems, emotions and thoughts. The therapeutic effect of dreaming, although it may make no sense in our waking hours, is vital for the general health of the body.

The average time people sleep is seven and a half hours, but statistically three hours on either side is within the normal range. As you grow older you need less sleep. Sleep problems can often be connected with nervous system depressants such as alcohol, barbiturates, opiates and benzodiazepine tranquillisers, for instance, Librium and Valium, as well as nervous system stimulants such as caffeine and amphetamines, medications for high blood pressure, hormones including thyroxine, cortisone and oral contraceptives, ulcer medications and anti-depressants. Excessive salt intake or nicotine can also affect sleeping patterns.

Helpful Non-herbal Aids for Relaxation

It is silly telling somebody to relax when they simply do not know how to, yet relaxation is possible and easy to learn. The choice of methods is wide and not all methods are suitable for every person. Relaxation methods include meditation, yoga, self-hypnosis, visualisation, autogenics and biofeedback. Sift through these until you find a method which is right for you and do not be discouraged because you are not instantly brilliant at it. Remember you almost certainly did not learn to read in a week. The secret is to persist with something you enjoy doing.

Experiments in America have proved that paradoxical intention is often very helpful for chronic insomniacs. This means doing the opposite of what you want to make happen. For instance, in one experiment, insomniacs were asked to stay awake as long as possible to note their insomniac thoughts and one woman reduced her wakeful period from ninety minutes to five and a half minutes!

Other things which may help include:

- Going to bed only when you are tired. Once in bed, do not watch the television, read or lie awake worrying. If you do not fall asleep quickly get up, go out of the bedroom and do something until you feel ready to try again.
- Set the alarm for the same time every morning, including weekends.
- Cut cigarettes, alcohol, stimulating drugs, refined carbohydrates and sugar out of your diet and eat a light supper.
- Exercising during the course of the day is of paramount importance. I have found that this is often the only regular tool an insomniac needs to use to ensure regular sleep. This should be done, if at all possible, outside. Have you ever noticed how a day spent outdoors makes you feel very tired when you return home?
- Alternative hot and cold showers, especially on the head, preceded by skin brushing also helps. However, I suggest you do not do either of these just before bed as they will act in the opposite way and keep you awake!
- Walking barefoot on soil or grass just before going to bed helps. I know it sounds crazy but what happens is that the excessive electrical charge built up in the body during the course of the day while walking on synthetic surfaces is released and literally grounded into the natural substance beneath your feet. Barefoot walking can be carried out for a minimum of five minutes on grass, sand or soil, after which the feet should be dried vigorously with a rough towel and then warm socks and shoes or slippers put on. This should be done just before going to bed. All you've got to risk is some funny looks from the neighbours!
- Alternatively, going to bed wearing a pair of loose-fitting wet cotton socks covered by a large pair of woollen socks is very helpful for inducing sleep. This doesn't feel as bad as it sounds.
- You should sleep in natural clothing, if you use any clothing at all, and in cotton sheets and the bed should be well aired. A healthy body will lose at least one and a half pints (0.75 litres) of fluid overnight into the surrounding material.
- Before going to bed take a bath at a temperature of 94–97°F with ten drops of lavender or chamomile oil added to your bath water. It will help to reduce congestion of the brain and spinal cord.
- Once in bed take ten to twenty slow, deep breaths of fresh air. This means you need to sleep with your window slightly ajar at night. If safety precautions preclude this, have an ioniser plugged in beside your bed at night.

Before going to bed take forty drops of anti-spasmodic tincture in warm water or drink two cups of the following tea:

Anti-spasmodic Tincture

Three parts:	hops
wood betony	lemon balm
One part:	vervain
catnip	chamomile

Infuse and sweeten if desired.

Alternatively, try Valerian tablets taken at the same time each night. Begin with one and increase the dose to two if necessary. They are extremely effective (see Resources Directory). Or you could try the nervine formulation on page 158.

INSECT STINGS

First remove the sting by flicking it out with your thumb nail so that the barb comes out cleanly without tearing the skin. If you have an ice-cube available rub it on the area; if not simply suck up and spit out the poisons. Rub tincture of plantain on to the skin or, if you do not have this, chew a plantain leaf into a pulp and apply it as a poultice over the sting, or apply a piece of raw onion to it. Take ten drops of plantain in water every two hours orally until the swelling and itching has subsided.

Stings in the throat

For insect stings in the throat, first gargle with four teaspoonfuls of salt in a cup of water and spit the gargle out. The salt water will draw out the poison. Then take ten drops of plantain in water every ten minutes orally and apply a cabbage leaf poultice externally to the neck.

Insect Repellents

To repel insects eat plenty of garlic or nutritional yeast.

Dr Christopher's Insect Repellent

Combine equal parts of rosemary, basil, wormwood and rue. Crush them together well in a pestle and mortar and pour over organic olive oil in proportions of one part of herbs to five parts of oil. Add one dessertspoonful of apple cider vinegar and cover the bowl. Set it over a radiator for a week. Strain well while the moisture is warm. Measure out the oil and repeat in proportions one part of fresh herbs added to five parts of the oil. Do this two more times and on the third occasion let the mixture sit over the radiator for at least two weeks. Strain well. You will now have an extremely effective concentrated oil which will keep insects away and is actually good for the skin at the same time. A little of it dabbed onto the insect sting will quickly help the swelling and itching go away.

To my mind this is far preferable to citronella oil in natural commercially marketed preparations. Citronella to me smells so nasty it acts as a human repellant not just an insect one!

ITCHING

Poisonous Plants

If the skin has been stung by a poisonous plant but there is no blistering, hold the area under running hot water at 120°F for a minute or so and then apply tincture of plantain.

Vulval itching

Vulval itching can be helped by a compress of goldenseal. As this stains everything bright yellow, remember to protect your underwear with a sanitary towel.

Rectal itching

Rectal itching, if it is not the result of bowel or rectal disease or antibiotics, can sometimes be the result of a poor reaction to coffee, tea, cold drinks, beer, chocolate or foods containing sugar or tomatoes. Take alternate hot and cold sitz-baths and apply tincture of goldenseal directly to the anal area. Alternatively, try garlic oil applied directly.

JET-LAG

Jet-lag only occurs when you cross one or more time zones and your body resists adjusting to new cycles of sleep and wakefulness. There is no jet-lag on north-south flights.

Adjust before you go

Begin to tackle this problem by adjusting as soon as you get on board the aeroplane. If, by your calculations, it will be night when you land, pull down the window blind, wear a sleep mask and try to sleep if possible. The remedies recommended for insomnia (see p. 191) which are easily portable, such as the anti-spasmodic drops and the nervine formulation, can be taken just before boarding the aircraft to assist sleep. If you fly at night and will be arriving during the day stay awake, keep your eyes open and the seat light on, trying to make sure that you are already in the new time zone. Reset your watch immediately after take-off because it will help you to get in tune with the new periods of day and night you will have to adjust to on arrival.

If you do land in daylight do not give in to the temptation to go to your hotel and crash out immediately. This will not only encourage your old rhythms to keep working, but will ensure that you take several days to get over your jet-lag. Stay outdoors if possible. If you are in a sunny country, sunlight will help because it stimulates the pineal and pituitary glands. So don't wear a hat or dark glasses when you get off the plane. If the weather keeps you indoors put the lights on and try to stay awake.

If you arrive at night go straight to your hotel room and sleep if you can.

Diet

Diet is helpful to some degree. For example, protein-rich foods can provide up to five hours of energy, whereas the foods that are high in carbohydrates such as pasta, salad, fruit and rich desserts provide an hour's energy surge but then tend to make you drowsy. If you arrive at your destination in the morning after a long flight and need to get down to work without delay, begin with a high protein breakfast and eat a high protein lunch to keep you going through the afternoon; for dinner eat carbohydrates to nurture sleep. A good high protein breakfast for a vegan could be nut milk or soya milk liquidised with fresh fruit, soya yogurt or a fruit smoothie with liberal amounts of spirulina added.

One of the habits that impedes recovery from jet-lag is eating meals at strange times. My husband and I generally find it better to fast and take lots of juices and still mineral water. I also travel with my own herbal tea bags and ask for hot water. The day after a long flight I eat as much fresh fruit as I can and if I am in a country where I suspect its cleanliness I choose thick-skinned fruit which needs peeling.

Aromatherapy

Daniele Ryman, one of our leading authorities on aromatherapy, sells an excellent set of essential oils to cope with jet-lag (see Resources Directory).

MISCARRIAGE

Most miscarriages occur during the first three months of pregnancy and many are caused by foetal abnormalities or defective implanting of the embryo in the womb. If there is any sign of a potential miscarriage get the mother to lie down immediately and take Rescue Remedy. **Meanwhile telephone the doctor**. Stay in bed and keep warm. Use a bed pan if necessary.

In my many years in clinical practice I have used Dr Christopher's miscarriage formulation dozens of times with success. The beauty of his combination of herbs is that they will not interfere with the natural process of miscarriage and if the foetus is damaged or dead the formulation will ease its expulsion.

I have also prevented many miscarriages with this formulation. I give women who are predisposed to miscarriage this formulation on standby.

Three parts of false unicorn root and one part of lobelia. Make a decoction and drink half a cup every half an hour. Once the bleeding stops, take it every hour for the rest of the day and then three times a day for the next three days. Lobelia is only available on prescription from qualified medical herbalists.

NIGHTMARES

Eat lightly before going to bed and combine foods correctly (see p. 32). Be sure that your colon is working properly and sip a cup of infused catnip tea with an individually selected Bach Flower remedy in it (see Resources Directory). Be selective about your daily mental input, including what you read, what you see, what you say and what you think. It all adds up.

NOSEBLEEDS

Squeeze the nose between the thumb and index finger just enough to stop the bleeding but not enough to make you wince. Breathe slowly through an open mouth, hold the pressure for a minimum of five minutes without stopping, then insert a ball of well-chewed yarrow leaf as high into each nostril as possible, but not so high it cannot be retrieved. Place the hands or feet in ice-cold water or put a bag of ice on the back of the neck. Often this alone will do the trick but if you are using the yarrow leaf continue to breathe through the mouth until your nose feels comfortable, then gently extract it.

Please note that if nosebleeds are frequent you must seek professional help.

POISONING

Above all keep the patient calm. Panic merely accelerates the speed with which the poison invades the system. **Seek immediate medical help**. Should the victim have swallowed a poisonous substance some hours before telephone the hospital immediately. If you don't know what the victim has swallowed and they are unable to tell you or are unconscious, describe the container and give all the information you can to the hospital over the phone. They will advise you what is to be done immediately while you wait for an ambulance.

Caustic poisoning

If the substance is caustic **do not** induce vomiting as it will only burn the throat further. **Seek immediate medical help.** Do not administer anything orally. Paracetamol does not induce a coma initially but in large quantities it can damage the liver, often fatally (see p. 202), so act quickly and get the victim to the hospital with the utmost speed.

FOOD POISONING

Follow the treatment recommended for diarrhoea (see p. 186); the stomach may be cleared by inducing vomiting with syrup of ipecacuana (see above)

Soothe the aching stomach afterwards with sips of very hot peppermint tea. Combat dehydration with plenty of fluids and chew as many charcoal tablets as possible. Ideally you should give twice the amount of charcoal as the suspected weight of the poison ingested. If you can get it, powdered charcoal, stirred into juice, is wonderful for absorbing any kind of toxic material in the gastro-intestinal tract.

SHOCK

I find Dr Bach's Rescue Remedy a supreme solution for this. The mother tincture should be diluted four drops in 2 fl oz (50 ml) of pure spring water to which you can add a little brandy as a preservative or, of you are allergic to alcohol, cider vinegar. Take four drops of this in one teaspoonful (5 ml) of water and hold it on the tongue for thirty seconds before swallowing. Repeat this at least four and up to six times daily. If the patient is unconscious, rub it into the lips or on the wrists (for suppliers see Resources Directory). Alternatively, take one teaspoonful of cayenne pepper in hot water or thirty drops of cayenne pepper in a little water. Continue to do this until normal colour returns and if necessary get medical help as quickly as possible.

My strong feeling is that the emotional affects of shock need to be helped immediately. If neglected they can reverberate through the system for years, causing an insidious build up of psychological and physiological problems.

SORE THROATS

See Coughs.

SPRAINS

If you have any doubt at all or think the joint may be fractured seek medical help. In the meantime apply an ice-pack to the area immediately. I have been known to use a packet of frozen peas in emergencies. If you need an ice-pack on an awkwardly shaped area, soak a towel in cold water, wring it out until it stops dripping and place it folded on foil in the freezer. Turn the freezer up to maximum. Leave the towel there until crystals form but it is not frozen solid. This way it will conform nicely to the injured area. If you need to massage an area with ice on a regular basis, fill a polystyrene or plastic cup with water and then freeze it. Once frozen, peel the cup to below ice level. This will give you a manageable block of ice and a cold-resistant handle. Keep the ice moving to avoid skin damage and stop the treatment the moment the skin becomes numb.

This type of massage has been found to be very useful in eighty per cent of patients complaining of chronic pain of various types ranging from lower back pain, rheumatoid and osteo-arthritis and cancer. It will supply relief for up to three hours.

As soon as the ice-pack is in place elevate the joint to stop effusion. If the fingers and toes turn blue you have overdone it. Once the swelling has reduced somewhat apply a compress of comfrey, securing it with a thin elasticated bandage. Leave this on for a day. Discourage moving, if at all possible. Do not walk on a sprained ankle. Use crutches if necessary. Enforce complete bed rest for back sprains and apply a sling to immobilise the sprain to a shoulder. If bruising is present once the swelling has subsided apply arnica tincture frequently.

SUNBURN

Patients have reported that Dr Christopher's insect repellent oil (see p. 191) makes a good sunburn treatment. Essential oil of lavender applied to severe sunburn on a dampened piece of gauze or muslin and left on as a poultice is very effective. This should be repeated every four hours.

STYES

Styes are usually a symptom of being extremely run down. If the stye is unbearably itchy, rub it with a piece of raw potato. Bathe the eyes with an infusion of marigold petals or a decoction of goldenseal. When you have time to rest try a warm compress of either of these herbs over a closed eyelid.

TOOTHACHE

First ensure that there is no impacted food around the aching tooth by using dental floss or a toothpick. Then apply an ice-pack against the jaw on the infected side. If you can see a cavity make sure it is clear by using a sterile cotton ball on the end of a toothpick, then pack into the hole a piece of crushed garlic or pour a small amount of oil of cloves into it.

If the hole is very large you may need to saturate a piece of cotton gauze with the oil of cloves first. Rub the surrounding gum with tincture of cayenne. Rub ice over the web of the skin between the thumb and index finger on the same side of the body as the pain is. This is not as daft as it sounds, this is the acupressure point used to relieve toothache. Naturally, make an appointment with your dentist as soon as possible.

TRAVEL SICKNESS

Simply chewing a piece of fresh ginger root or taking some powdered ginger has proved to be twice as effective for travel sickness as some over-the-counter remedies.

I am prone to almost every type of travel sickness there is and I have found an acupressure point called *Nei-Kuan* which helps to relieve all sorts of sickness. It can be found on the surface of the inside of both forearms three fingers widths away from the crease of the wrist and in the centre between the two flex tendons. Press this point with the tip of the thumb firmly (obviously short finger nails help here) and repeat as often as necessary. A specially designed wrist strap with a rounded plastic button that will do this for you is available through pharmacists.

I have found that it also helps to focus on distant objects while travelling in a car or on a train, rather than on nearby ones moving fast. My favourite seat on a plane is over the wheels, rather than in the tail which moves more than the rest of the aircraft. On a ship I try to stay on deck as much as I can, no matter what the weather. Gusts of fresh air and sea spray keep my mind focused on better things!

APPENDIX 1

——

Since the turn of the century the drug industry has grown into one of the largest industries in the world. The USA recognised the importance of this industry and the need for tight controls by the Food and Drug Administration (FDA). The FDA publishes, as a matter of course, its reasons for granting a licence to a drug and how the decisions are arrived at.

However, in the UK the British drug industry argues against this type of control on the grounds of cost. The UK Medicines Control Agency (MCA) is responsible for the licensing of new drugs and is entirely funded by applications from the drug companies.

On top of this the drug companies maintain a level of secrecy which almost borders on fanaticism. The drug industry, with the tacit agreement of the British government, is entitled to withhold vital evidence regarding the dangers of drugs. It is alleged that the resource and testing of new drugs is not always as thorough as the public has a right to expect and there have been examples of drug trials being falsified.

The findings of the FDA are available to the general public through a massive book known as the *Physicians' Desk Reference*. This book gives details of every available drug and any risks that may be involved in the use thereof. To date over 30 million copies have been sold. In the UK we have a much smaller reference book known as MIMS. This covers only a selection of drugs and is very selective when it comes to dealing with any possible dangers or side-effects.

In money the ratio spent in marketing drugs as opposed to offering information about them stands at 40:1. The MCA is the **only** drugs agency in the EC which is so utterly dependent on the potential licensee. Our system of drug regulations is in need of an overhaul.

Here is a brief reference to some of the most common drugs the women I work with ask me about. It is by no means complete. It is simply a start. If you want to know more contact:

- **The U.S. Food and Drug Administration**
  Anyone, in any country, has the right to ask for information about drugs licensed by the FDA, courtesy of the American Freedom of Information Act. Begin by writing a letter to the FDA, Freedom of Information Office, 5600 Fishers Lane, Rockville, MD 20857. They are legally obliged to respond within ten days if only to say that your request is being

investigated. When you write ask for the Summary Basis of Approval (SBA) on the drugs that concern you, making sure to find out the American generic and brand name first, as drug names are different in some countries. The SBA will include a detailed summary of appropriate information including the results of clinical trials that formed the basis of the FDA's decision to approve that drug. You should also ask for Adverse Drug Reactions (ADRs). These are unverified reports of any side-effects reported and they include MedWatch Reports (this is the new database of Drug Reactions recently set up by the FDA).

Payment* is $3 per request and after the first 100 pages of photocopying and the first two hours of research, which are free, you will be charged ten cents for each page of photocopying and a fee varying between $13 and $46 an hour. This is dependent upon the grade level of the person required to do the research. By all means ask for an estimate of how much your search will cost in your initial letter. *Payment is correct at time of press.

- Alternatively, try the Science reference section of any large library. There you should find the *American Physicians' Desk Reference* or the ABPI's *Data Sheet Compendium* on the shelf which you can use to look up anything you need to know.

- Or you could visit a large medical book shop. They tend to have quite a few useful volumes about drugs. I brought my own *PDR* across from America, but if you are asking friends to do this for you be aware of the fact that it is a huge volume. The UK *Data Sheet Compendium* can be ordered from the British Medical Journal book shop in Tavistock Square, London WC1, telephone 0171 387 4499 or directly from ABPI at Datapharm Publications, 12 Whitehall, London SW1, telephone 0171 930 3477. At the time of press it costs £32 inclusive of postage
- You could also investigate a drug industry magazine called, appropriately enough, *Scrip*. It is possible to buy back issues for £5 each. Not only does it report on all the new information that has emerged about drug side-effects but it receives SBA's regularly. Write to 18–20 Hill Rise, Richmond, Surrey, TW10 6UA, or telephone 0181 948 3262.
- In addition to all of this, I would urge you to subscribe to an excellent newsletter called *What Doctors Don't Tell You*. The guidance I have just given you is pioneered by them in their excellent and determined campaign to stop drug secrecy. *WDDTY* sends out a twelve-page newsletter monthly which, since 1989, has covered most major health issues. It also publishes various excellent handbooks and filofax guides and, in my opinion, is well researched, pugnacious and courageously outspoken. It is worth every penny of the yearly subscription. Write to *What Doctors Don't Tell You*, 4 Wallace Road, London, N1 2PG.

• ANTIBIOTICS •

Research confirms that antibiotics are massively and incorrectly used for conditions they simply cannot treat, especially ear, nose and throat problems, viral infections and cystitis. For example, in only half of all the so-called cases of cystitis is E. coli bacteria (the true cause of cystitis) actually present. Hospitals tend to use antibiotics on a 'just in case' basis for clean surgeries like hysterectomies and appendectomies which shouldn't need them. I think doctors use a blunderbuss approach with broad spectrum antibiotics that kill all bacteria, even the friendly kind. Imipenem is a case in point.

However, antibiotics disturb the friendly bacteria that live in and around the body resulting in digestive problems like diarrhoea, constipation and nausea and they may even provoke life-threatening colitis or diverticulitis in the elderly. The poisons that ferment as a result of the putrefying bacteria that take over can cause headaches, fatigue, confusion and insomnia. Antibiotics can also create holes in the intestinal walls through which poisons can seep into the body, resulting in allergies and the loss of nutrients. This is particularly true of fungal infections like candida. Recent research has suggested that this intestinal porosity can cause eczema and allergies and there is now some suggestion that it may lead to Crohn's disease and irritable bowel syndrome (IBS).

Certain antibiotics present specific problems. Chloramphenicol has been known to cause aplastic anaemia in one in 20,000 cases, yet astonishingly it is still available over the counter without a prescription in certain countries and is certainly over-used in the UK and the USA. Erythromycin esolate is recorded as causing liver damage and abdominal pain in one in 100 people. It is banned in the USA but not yet in the UK. Sulphonamides, though now considered a bit old fashioned, and trimethoprim can cause rashes and allergic reactions and can damage the kidneys by forming crystals in them. Hopefully, most doctors are now aware that sulphonamides can cause a dangerous bone marrow disease and consequently harm the foetus in pregnant women. Gentamycin and neomycin cause deafness in one in 100 people and I have personally witnessed allergic reactions (anaphylaxis, that is immediate shock or delayed shock) in patients. It accounts for ten per cent of all reactions to antibiotics and can be fatal in one in 50,000 people.

Besides all this, **antibiotics are suppressive**, stopping the body from fighting the infection properly and leaving it with unhealed residues which can cause much more serious problems later in life. Repeated courses of antibiotics merely encourage supergerms. This can affect the public at large as it has done with gonorrhoea, for example, and staphylococcus infections, which now need to be treated with massive courses of antibiotics, where two or three decades ago a normal course of penicillin would do.

But what is most worrying to me is that repeated courses of antibiotics appear to disturb the immune system in ways medicine has yet to divine.

I would recommend that you do not take antibiotics for:

- viral infections like colds, flu and sore throats and gastro-enteritis;
- mastitis;
- cystitis;

- Athlete's foot (which is a fungus);
- infection-caused fever, which is simply nature's efficient way of killing the offending organism. Dehydration is the main concern with fevers less than three days old, so what I would prescribe is rest, warmth and lots of juices and herbal teas to encourage the fever. Remember the classic one of equal parts of peppermint, elderflower and yarrow. A more pleasant tea is ginger with plenty of honey and lemon in it. Remember to drink a lot of purified water.

To counteract the effect of any antibiotics take a course of bioacidophilus which will ensure candida and fungus don't overwhelm your digestive tract. Alternatively, remember the king of herbs, garlic, which is one of the few herbs capable of repopulating the benign flora in your gut. Enjoy those immune boosters of sunlight, hydrotherapy, gentle lymphatic pumping exercise and skin brushing. Bear in mind that extra manganese in the diet is needed to counteract the damaging effect of neomycin (this is available in sprouted wheat, wheatgerm and seeds). Extra vitamin E (found in the same foods) helps to prevent the liver toxicity produced by tetracyclines. Liver flushes will also help (see p. 63).

• ASPIRIN, PARACETAMOL, IBUPROFEN AND OTHER PAINKILLING DRUGS •

ASPIRIN

As you get to this section I can almost hear you groaning, 'Leave good old aspirin alone, surely that can't be harmful!'

Many people don't think of aspirin as a drug simply because it has been available since 1899 and marketed in its current form for more than eighty years. But were it to be subjected to FDA investigation today it would certainly not get a licence.

Aspirin interferes with a series of chemicals in our bodies called prostaglandins, inhibiting some of them, then raising the temperature of the body. Prostaglandins also play a major part in creating inflammation in the body so while aspirins are prescribed for inflammation of the joints they are also widely used to interfere with blood clotting and are often thought of as blood thinners, although this is not quite accurate. In fact it will take **longer** for bleeding to stop after aspirin has been swallowed because of the affect it has on platelets, a key component of blood clotting. One adult aspirin will permanently inactivate all the platelets in the blood for some considerable time, and remember there are millions of them. Only a fraction of an adult aspirin, about one-tenth, is needed to deactivate all the platelets in circulation in the bloodstream at any one time. Now these platelets are constantly being replenished by the bone marrow, from which all the blood cells are produced. They survive between ten and fourteen days within the circulatory system and every day we lose approximately ten per cent of them. The newly released platelets are not affected by a dose of aspirin given the day before, only by aspirin taken on the same day. This is the reason why doctors ask patients **not** to take any aspirin for at least one week before surgery, because just one aspirin taken close to an operation may result in intra-operative bleeding and increase the likelihood of the patient needing a blood transfusion.

Among other things, aspirin is a severe stomach irritant. It can cause erosions, ulcers and gastro-enteritis, all of which can result in internal bleeding. But as I have already pointed out, aspirin also inhibits blood clotting, so when stomach bleeding occurs it is difficult for the body to control it. The dosage of aspirin recommended in the *Physicians' Desk Reference* is up to 4,000 mg a day but studies of its side-effects cite 'gross intestinal bleeding which is clinically significant, vomiting blood and stomach pain', and this can be caused by doses of only 1,000 mg which is three ordinary adult aspirins daily. Yet the *PDR* would have you taking two tablets every four hours! In fact hospitalisation for gastro-intestinal disorders is forty per cent higher for aspirin users. In addition, aspirin can cause bleeding which is independent of the dose. The effect on platelets caused by only one aspirin results in a sluggish ability to form blood clots and in some people this can contribute to significant bleeding, particularly in the brain. I have known some of my patients to be anaemic simply because they were losing a lot of blood from taking aspirin. If you simply must take aspirin (although there are a number of harmless and positively beneficial alternatives, such as meadowsweet, valerian, chamomile and white willow bark) take them with a drink of slippery elm or marshmallow root to soothe and protect the stomach lining.

There are also vitamin losses produced by aspirin. Extra B vitamins and vitamin C help to protect the adrenal glands from being overstimulated by aspirin and so protect the kidneys.

Aspirin can cause temporary infertility as well as loss of hearing and tinnitus. It has also been known to cause allergies, swollen lymph nodes, generalised swelling, drops in blood pressure, breathing problems, diarrhoea, nasal polyps and hives. **Flu and chicken pox should never be treated by aspirin.** Such treatment may cause Reye's syndrome, which can be fatal. Remember any process which can be exacerbated by bleeding, including dental surgery and childbirth, precludes the use of aspirin.

The now popular and widespread use of aspirin to prevent strokes is **not** supported by the scientific evidence. Of sixteen studies that have recently taken place, all have proved to be flawed one way or another. Only one of the studies met the criteria of a properly designed clinical trial!

PARACETAMOL

If paracetamol was applying for a licence today, like aspirin, it would never be allowed for sale without a prescription. Paracetamol has an extremely destructive effect on the liver. The problem is that the liver is one of the two key organs, together with the kidneys, which disposes of chemical drugs. It can cope with the recommended dose of paracetamol but if too much is taken all the glutathione is used up. Without this protective factor paracetamol goes on a destructive rampage destroying liver tissue. Parasuicides are treated in hospital with cystein which creates more glutathione. If you must take paracetamol I recommend you support the liver by taking foods rich in selenium, vitamin C and vitamin E. They are rich in antioxidants which stabilise levels of glutathione in the liver. Garlic is particularly rich in selenium and has been proved to protect the liver from damage by chemicals. To a lesser extent so do onions, ginger, radish and horseradish.

The recommended maximum dose of paracetamol is 49 grams a day. A dose of 6.39 grams a day has been found to be toxic to the liver and paracetamol is one of the commonest causes of liver failure. Combined with aspirin it is much more toxic than if either drug were taken alone; it can also harm the kidneys. If you have to make a choice aspirin is safer than paracetamol, which in turn is safer than ibuprofen (see the following section). All sorts of excellent alternative ways of coping with pain, both mental and physical, have been described throughout this book.

• NON-STEROID ANTI-INFLAMMATORY DRUGS (NSAIDS) •

Unlike steroids these do not act on the adrenal hormones, but on local hormones called prostaglandins which play a major part in creating inflammation in the body. They are widely prescribed for any sort of pain as the result of inflammation, particularly for arthritis and occasionally for dysmenorrhoea. They affect the kidneys by blocking the prostaglandins there, and can lead to kidney failure, fluid retention in the arms and legs and, as a result, a sodium-potassium imbalance in the body, gastro-intestinal upsets and bleeding, hair and fingernail loss, loss of appetite, fevers, dizziness, insomnia, depression, epilepsy, Parkinson's disease, double vision or blurring of vision, hearing loss and tinnitus, asthma and breathing difficulties, alterations in blood pressure and cardiac arrhythmias, and chest pains. The effect of these drugs on the kidneys is particularly worrying because they are thought to cause the tiny tubes in the kidneys to degenerate, reducing the function of them more or less permanently. If there are any pre-existing kidney or heart problems, these drugs can cause further disturbances on these organs. There is also a three to four times greater risk of kidney cancer as a result of the effect of stripping the lining of the stomach which I have previously noted. This relentless degeneration can lead to holes through which unwanted material can filter and in turn creates allergies. People using them long term need to have hearing and eye tests on a regular basis as well as frequent renal and hepatic functional tests and blood counts.

HERBAL HELP

Vitamin E reduces the kidney damage caused by these drugs and can prevent scarring there. The dose needs to be built up gradually especially for those who have any blood pressure problems. I have found herbs rich in gamma linolenic acid (GLA) very helpful when I have been weaning patients off these drugs, particularly in view of the fact that GLA is one of the natural components of the prostaglandin chain that appears to be disturbed or deficient in arthritis and other inflammatory diseases.

GLA is richly present in evening primrose oil and blackcurrant seed oil. Aloe vera juice, when swallowed, is wonderful for inflammation of the intestines and stomach pain inflammation as the result of these drugs. To a limited degree it helps stop allergic reactions created by drugs, yeasts or penetration of the stomach lining. But the tool that I found the most effective to help heal inflammation in any part of the body is controlled fasting. This, coupled with anti-inflammatory and blood cleansing herbs, is wonderfully effective.

In my experience all types of rheumatic disease are greatly helped by alkaline diets. The ideal alkaline diet is a vegan one because it excludes acid foods such as meat, fish, dairy products, eggs, caffeinated drinks and anything refined.

IBUPROFEN

As for ibuprofen, one of the most popular NSAIDs, the *Physicians' Desk Reference* warns that it can cause 'severe gastro-intestinal bleeding, ulceration and perforation'. The worrying thing is this can occur without any warning whatsoever. The *PDR* also cites dyspepsia as common with the usage of this drug. Moreover, one out of six people taking it have an adverse reaction; one out of twenty-five who use it for a year get upper gastro-intestinal ulcers and growths, bleeding or perforation, requiring hospitalisation. Cases of death have been reported as a result. Other problems as the result of taking ibuprofen include severe hepatic reactions, jaundice, fatal hepatitis, a decrease in the haemoglobin, aseptic meningitis, fever, coma, renal papillary necrosis and nephritis. In the long run I am afraid that ibuprofen will be proved to be even more damaging than aspirin.

• BLOOD PRESSURE DRUGS •

Many people prescribed blood pressure drugs think they have to take them for life. They seem to be incapable of exploring the reasons why they have blood pressure and dealing with those, rather than treating the symptoms with drugs which have a plethora of side-effects including impotence, headache, weakness, depression, dizziness, dry mouth, rash, constipation, insomnia and nausea.

Moreover, it can be dangerous to stop taking high blood pressure drugs abruptly once on them because they can induce a rebound effect in which the blood pressure can shoot sky high leading to stroke and death. If this weren't bad enough, reserpine is still prescribed for high blood pressure even though it was discovered in 1974 to **triple** the risk of breast cancer.

BETABLOCKERS

Betablocking agents such as Netoprolol tartare USP, commonly known as Lopressor, are widely prescribed for treating hypertension. However, according to the *PDR* 'the mechanism of the anti-hypertensive effect of betablocking agents has not been elucidated'. This kind of information is constantly echoed throughout the PDR and I find it interesting, particularly because medical herbalists are frequently rebuked by allopaths for not understanding how their herbal medication works, once ingested! Besides the pharmacological research that is being done into herbal medicine all over the world, we also have thousands of years of empirical experience with our medicines. Synthetic drugs can't match this and pharmacologists privately admit mystification as to their mechanics.

As far as Lopressor is concerned, the PDR warns of a continued depression of the myocardium with betablocking agents over a period of time, which can lead to cardiac failure. It goes on to say, 'if cardiac failure is present, Lopressor should be withdrawn . . . following abrupt cessation of therapy with betablocking agents, myocardial infarction can occur'. What this means is that if you have high blood pressure and are afraid this could cause a stroke or heart attack you take Lopressor to lower your blood pressure, but its continued use can cause a heart attack, in which case you should stop using it immediately, but stopping it abruptly can give you a heart attack! An amazing catch-twenty-two situation! If your heart stops as a result of withdrawal from Lopressor, the medics could have difficulty in restarting and maintaining the heartbeat. This has been reported on several occasions with patients who use betablockers.

Another commonly used betablocker is verapamil hydrochloride, which is a calcium iron influx inhibitor (a slow-channel blocker or calcium iron antagonist). This is generally used to reduce high blood pressure and relieve angina but the warning in the PDR states that two per cent of patients develop congestive heart failure or pulmonary oedema and several cases of liver damage have been proven.

ADVERSE REACTIONS

Adverse reactions from betablockers include bronchial spasm, tiredness, dizziness, depression, mental confusion, memory loss, headache, nightmares, insomnia, diarrhoea, nausea, abdominal pain, rashes, psoriasis, diabetes, mental depression leading to catatonia, clouded senses, fever, sore throat, respiratory distress and hypertension. Severe cases of overdose leading to death have been reported and frighteningly there is no specific antidote.

The diuretics commonly used to remove excess body water to assist high blood pressure can harm the kidneys and cause or worsen diabetes. They can produce nausea, stomach and digestive problems, dizziness, headache, tinnitus and bone problems.

FINDINGS

The statistic that causes me concern is that three-quarters of the patients who have been on these blood pressure-lowering drugs do not even need them! A $150 million study in the United States showed that those treated with drugs for high blood pressure tended to have a higher death rate than any other group. A similar but much smaller twelve-year study in the UK run by the Medical Research Council, found that drug treatment for hypertension **did not save lives or reduce the risk of heart attacks**. The study found that twenty per cent of the patients had side-effects including impotence, pre-diabetes and gout, and these unfortunate patients withdrew from the study. The study finally advised that these drugs only be used to treat high blood pressure in very severe cases.

Of course naturopaths and medical herbalists have known for very many decades that a non-pharmacological approach to raised blood pressure is far preferable and we use all sorts of means including reduced weight, if this is necessary, reduced dietary salt intake, more exercise, relaxation, visualisation and meditation techniques, general dietary management especially Superfoods and juices, and of course herbs.

● CORTICOSTEROIDS ●

Corticosteroids are generally used to treat allergies, inflammation, endocrine disorders, diseases with no recognised cause or due to autoimmune factors and rheumatic problems, and were once touted as miracle drugs. But the truth is now out. The FDA has come clean and warns the public, 'Many patients quickly reverted to their previous condition when cortisone treatment ceased. And, even worse, devastating and frightening side-effects often accompanied cortisone treatment . . . Side-effects included insomnia, psychotic behaviour, growth suppression in children, peptic ulcer, delayed wound healing, hyperglycaemia, carbohydrate intolerance, muscle weakness, susceptibility to infections and many others'. Coming from the FDA, which is notoriously conservative and drug-orientated, this is enough to make anyone take a deep breath and pause for thought.

Surgeons have reported death under general anaesthesia of people undergoing relatively minor surgery who have been taking cortisones. Perhaps one of the most insidious things of all is that cortisone is habit forming and stopping it often produces painful withdrawal symptoms.

Steroids can also cause cataracts or damage the optic nerve, affect fat metabolism, cause osteoporosis, thin skin, and ultimately cause massive chemical imbalance in the body, resulting in death during stressful situations. They have been proven to cause hypoadrenalism in babies born of mothers taking steroids.

The only instance in which I can think of steroids being justified is to treat shock from allergic reactions or serious injuries on an extremely temporary basis, but steroids are still used to treat asthma, allergies, rheumatic disorders, eczema and other skin diseases and colitis. In all these cases, steroids suppress the symptoms but the disease still remains deeply entrenched with increasingly horrific side-effects.

The problem is by the time patients consult me after prolonged ingestion of steroids I can't simply manufacture a new adrenal gland for them. However, there are herbs and dietary managements that can greatly help over a period of time if the patient is prepared to be very persistent. But management needs to be followed under the close supervision of a good naturopath or herbalist experienced in this field and, most importantly, steroids need to be tapered off very gradually indeed, not simply because of the horrific physical toll they rap on the body but because of the psychological ones including nervousness, insomnia, mood swings ranging from mania to depression, disorientation, apathy and memory loss.

• CHOLESTEROL-REDUCING DRUGS

Atherosclerosis, which accounts for ninety-nine per cent of coronary artery disease, develops when the cholesterol in the bloodstream deposits sludge inside the lining of the arteries; this is difficult to do because every artery has a natural protective barrier. Cholesterol first has to seep through that barrier before it can stick and the process is generally a very slow one. The level of cholesterol, while important in predicting heart disease, is not the entire story. There are those with the in-built ability to resist high cholesterol levels, perhaps because they are born with a stronger protective barrier and are less vulnerable to the penetration of cholesterol, and these differences are often hereditary. There are others less fortunate who are particularly predisposed to congestion with cholesterol. I am able to detect whether a person has such a familial tendency to producing too much cholesterol by observing a lipemic diathesis in the iris during the course of an iridology test.

Interestingly, research has shown that a diet of less than ten per cent fat works very much better to reduce cholesterol levels than cholesterol-lowering drugs. Clofibrates like Atromind-S have been in use for some time and yet the *PDR* admits 'The mechanism of its action has not been established definitely'. It may inhibit the hepatic release of lipoproteins but nobody knows for certain. Side-effects can include fatigue, weakness, headache, dizziness, muscle ache, hair loss, drowsiness, tremors, blurred vision, perspiration, impotence, decreased sex drive, anaemia, peptic ulcer, rheumatoid arthritis and lupus erythenatosis. The *PDR* states 'It has not been established whether drug-induced lowering of cholesterol is detrimental, beneficial or has no effect on the morbidity or mortality due to atherosclerotic coronary heart disease. Several years will be required before scientific investigation will yield the answer to this question . . . In a large study involving 10,000 patients – 5,000 on clofibrate, 5,000 on placebos for six years (also linked with a World Health Organisation study) – **The group on clofibrate had a thirty-five per cent higher death rate due to non-cardiovascular causes**' (my emphasis). Half the deaths were due to cancer, the other half due to complications after the necessary removal of the gall-bladder. Very often the cancer was due to pancreatic disease. In other words what this drug does is hold fats in the liver, refusing to let them into the bloodstream, so the liver becomes toxic and congested. After some time the drug taker will inevitably reap the consequences.

DIETARY MANAGEMENT

Dietary management including fasting can reduce your cholesterol levels in a matter of weeks and I have proved this over and over again in my extensive work with patients with high cholesterol levels. Such an approach avoids unpleasant side-effects including muscle cramps, tenderness and stiffness, severe stomach pains, nausea and vomiting and a skin rash. If I haven't yet managed to put you off, a further warning, do not take cholesterol-reducing drugs if you are pregnant, have kidney or liver disease, gall-bladder disease or gall-stones. Remember to take extra vitamin A and D since these drugs interfere with the absorption of both these vitamins, which are richly present in many of the superfoods (see pp.25–32) as well as carrot juice.

• TRANQUILLISERS AND SLEEPING PILLS •

Benzodiazepines, the most notorious being Valium and Ativan, were introduced in the 1960s as a supposedly safer alternative to the acknowledged habit-forming barbiturates and since then have become the most widely prescribed drugs in the world. Fifteen per cent of people living in first world countries take them every year and dependence on tranquillisers is much more common among women than men. Doctors prescribe them for anxiety, depression, agoraphobia and insomnia, and despite the recommendation of the Committee on Safety of Medicines that they should only be taken for between two and four weeks, three and a half million Britons have taken tranquillisers for more than four months; such chronic over-usage is commoner among the elderly and women. The problem is as bad in the USA. The Health Research Group in America logged almost one-fifth of all Americans over 65 as being on tranquillisers and eleven per cent on hypnotics for at least a year. Three-quarters of all these people were women.

SIDE-EFFECTS

The terrifying thing is there is no evidence that there is any benefit in taking tranquillisers and sleeping pills over any length of time. Counselling is at least as effective, if not more so. Indeed some of these drugs actually **increase** the very symptoms they are supposed to alleviate. Depression and anxiety can be caused by tranquillisers. They can cause drowsiness and confusion and should never be taken with alcohol or while driving. They can cause birth defects and problems for a baby if taken during the last three months of pregnancy or when breastfeeding, so they should not be taken if you are pregnant. Nor should they be taken if you have kidney or liver disease, or respiratory disease such as chronic bronchitis or emphysema, as one of the side-effects is difficulty with breathing.

They have also been observed to cause anger, rage, hostility, trembling, fear, apprehension, insomnia, nightmares and suicidal tendencies. Some baby battering has been linked to the taking of tranquillisers.

There have even been suggestions that they may assist the growth and spread of an already existent cancer. (Certainly changes in white blood cells have been recorded.) They can cause visual disturbances including delirium and hallucination as well as hearing difficulties, rashes, excitement, sexual fantasies, difficulty in walking, falling and fractures. Of the 227,000 hip fractures that take place in America every year, almost exclusively in older people, some 10,000 are directly linked to the use of sleeping pills or tranquillisers. Whereas a younger person may ride through such an accident easily, it can be life threatening for an older one.

WITHDRAWAL

Benzodiazepines are now acknowledged to be highly addictive and there are those who feel Ativan is so addictive it ought to be banned. I have assisted many women off both tranquillisers and sleeping pills with herbs, nutritional support, hydro-therapy including essential oils, counselling, aromatherapy, acupressure and exercise, but herbs should **never** be used as substitutes and withdrawal needs to be slow and carefully controlled by a professional medical herbalist with experience in this field. Much depends on my bond with the patient, but I normally don't start dropping the dose of the tranquillisers or sleeping pills for the first five days, then I ease it down by a fifth every week, adjusting my herbal medication to alleviate any differing symptoms that may arise.

• DRUGS TO TREAT DEPRESSION •

TRICYCLIC ANTI-DEPRESSANTS

If the depression is not endogenous the cause should always be addressed and although it generally comes down to stress from various sources (marital, divorce, bereavement or unemployment) physical causes should also be investigated, including thyroid insufficiency, hypoglycaemia, poor diet and, of course, side-effects from other drugs. Other factors inducing depression can include certain cancers (bowel, lymph node, brain or pancreatic), although having cancer in itself would naturally be very depressing, hepatitis or viral pneumonias, strokes, Parkinson's or Alzheimer's disease. With specific reference to Parkinson's, both the illness and so-called cure of anti-parkinsonian drugs can induce depression.

The physical structure of wheat has been altered markedly over the last 150 years and in my experience it is one of the commonest food intolerances as far as adults are concerned. Whilst sprouted wheat is perfectly acceptable I have often found it necessary to move patients over to alternative grains for bread. Severe vitamin C deficiency can also manifest as depression, as can deficiencies of B-complex vitamins and various minerals.

SIDE-EFFECTS

Very severe depression does need rapid intervention but tricyclics should be an absolute last resort because the side-effects can be worse than the problem itself. They include confusion and short-term memory problems, a disturbed attention span, dizziness, drowsiness, delirium, disorientation, fatigue, blurred vision, difficulty in urinating, constipation, sleepiness, the worsening of glaucoma, a dangerous plunge in blood pressure levels and heart rhythm disturbances including heart attacks, excessive sweating and, not surprisingly given this horrific list, sexual dysfunction. The tricyclics can also lead to rapid weight gain. In a recent study of ninety-three patients given these drugs, thirty-one per cent began to eat excessively and become overweight and thirty-four per cent had an insatiable craving for sugar.

PROZAC

Prozac was launched four years ago and lauded in the media as a breakthrough in the treatment of depression. Now numerous prozac users are in the middle of suing Lilly, the pharmaceutical company that manufacture it, claiming that the drug causes suicidal and homicidal thoughts and actions. Lilly themselves have admitted that up to fifteen per cent of patients in initial clinical trials reported anxiety and insomnia and some patients reported significant weight loss and even anorexia. Prozac's side-effects include visual disturbances, hypomania, trembling and palpitations, flu-like symptoms, rapid heartbeat, back pain, rashes, sweating, nausea, diarrhoea, abdominal pain, loss of libido, double vision, memory loss, cataracts or glaucoma, asthma, arthritis, osteoporosis, bleeding from the stomach wall, kidney inflammation and antisocial behaviour. As a prozac user in the United States killed five and wounded twelve others at the printing plant where he worked I would certainly concur that that is antisocial behaviour!

Prozac should definitely not be taken with other psycho-active drugs. It increases the action of warfarin, digoxin and it prolongs the effects of benzodiazepines. Those taking prozac with tryptophan can become upset with painful stomachs.

Rapid withdrawal from any of these drugs is not recommended and the symptoms of withdrawal can be much more severe than those of tranquillisers.

Indeed depression can return re-doubled. Please note all anti-depressants react with alcohol, street drugs including cocaine, general anaesthetic and painkillers. This is only the thin edge of the wedge as many drugs cause depression as one of their side-effects so if your last resort is to take anti-depressants please **never** take them without a thorough evaluation. Do not use them if you have glaucoma, any heart problems or difficulties with blood pressure (indeed you are advised to take an electro-cardiogram before starting these drugs), particularly if you have any cardiovascular problems or are on drugs for high blood pressure. They should not be married with tranquillisers, stimulants, sleeping pills, alcohol, anti-histamines or thyroid drugs. You need to wait at least two weeks after stopping these drugs before embarking on MAOI anti-depressants.

HERBAL HELP

Again I have found specific herbs coupled with counselling very effective as a means of weaning people off anti-depressants and interestingly enough skin brushing coupled with manual lymphatic drainage or aromatherapy has also proved extremely useful, I suspect, because all of these stimulate the glandular system at a very profound level.

• FEMALE SEX HORMONES •

SYNTHETIC OESTROGEN INCLUDING THE PILL

I am planning to write a book about the wrong thinking behind these because the catalogue of problems associated with them is so vast. Dr Helen Grant in her excellent book, *The Bitter Pill* states that the Pill is 'the most powerful immune suppressant known in medicine'. Her evidence of the Pill's effects on almost every system in the body is so vast that I am unable to list it here but it includes blood clots, disturbances in vision, blindness, increased risk of birth defects, strokes, slurred speech, mental depression, migraines, heart attack, thromboembolism as well as, most worryingly of all, breast, cervical, uterine and liver cancers. Her findings have been endorsed by an increasing number of recent studies.

CANCER

'The standardised incidence rate for cervical cancer in women who had taken the Pill for more than ten years was four times that in never-users.' Hitherto, the terrible increase in cervical cancer had been dumped on sexual activity. The sadness is so much emphasis has been placed by the media on greater sexual activity including numbers of partners and sexually transmitted disease that women with cervical cancer tended to be reluctant to speak out about their diagnosis to those close to them.

Women under forty who have never had a full-term pregnancy and who have taken the Pill for ten years or more are four times as likely to get breast cancer than non-Pill users. Those who have taken the Pill for a shorter period of time, for four to eight years, run an increased risk of forty per cent of developing breast cancer by the time they are in their mid-thirties. This escalates to seventy per cent if they have been taking the Pill for more than eight years. (For alternative methods of contraception see pp.118–19.)

• HORMONE REPLACEMENT THERAPY (HRT) •

The fact that Premarin is manufactured, in my opinion, cruelly, from the urine of pregnant mares, seems to me enough to make any right thinking person draw breath and pause before submitting to the medical profession's concept of the menopause as a deficiency disease. I am absolutely certain that the prolonged experiment carried out by the Pill and HRT on women this century will prove to be medicine's biggest and costliest mistake. HRT is usually a combination of oestrogen and progesterone, similar in make up to the Pill, although some contraceptive Pills are made from progesterone only.

HRT AND OSTEOPOROSIS

Far from preventing osteoporosis, HRT actually precipitates it. Of 670 women studied in Massachusetts, 112 were on oestrogen therapy. The conclusion? That HRT preserves bone mass **only when it is taken for upwards of seven years**; as soon as HRT was stopped bone mineral density declined rapidly. In women aged seventy-five, it was 3.2 per cent higher than in those women who had never taken oestrogen. In a study carried out at the Nuffield Orthopaedic Centre at Oxford over fifty per cent of the bone density of rabbits was lost by administering oestrogen and cortisols (the latter used to represent the effects of daily stress). Not that I approve of any studies conducted on animals but the researcher who carried this out said 'as a direct action of corticosteroids on removing bone, that includes all but one of the main progestogen compounds, and if you alternate it with oestrogen there is more bone loss than with oestrogen alone'.

The most remarkable thing about osteoporosis and HRT is that the average woman has her menopause in her fifties but the greatest risk of hip fractures occurs in her seventies, eighties or nineties. So HRT in this respect can hardly be said to be protecting women from osteoporosis.

HRT AND OTHER DISEASES

Besides this HRT trebles the risk of endometrical cancer and quadruples the risk of breast cancer. In 1991 an updated review in the USA of the evidence of HRT's reported protective effects against cardiovascular disease proved to be similarly flawed. Indeed there is some evidence that the risk of heart disease with users of HRT may actually be **increased**.

Nor does HRT protect you from dementia, forgetfulness or strokes in old age. There is also growing evidence that oestrogen implants and, to a lesser degree, patches are psychologically as well as physically addictive.

Pharmaceutical companies maintain that the 'natural' oestrogens (remember where it comes from!) of HRT don't have the same risk of thrombosis as the Pill but a study of sixty women on a continuous oestrogen-progestogen combination showed changes in blood coagulation and the ability of the body to break up clots. Two of these women developed thrombosis.

Progesterones can also alter glucose and insulin levels, cause higher than normal levels of calcium, hepatitis, liver cancer, jaundice, excess fluid and an increase in facial hair as well as the deepening of the voice (the last two can be irreversible). Because of over stimulation of the vascular system it can cause migraines or increase their severity. Other studies suggest that HRT makes endometriosis much worse and accelerates the chances of cystitis. So do not take HRT if you have a history of breast cancer in the family, any problems with blood clot formation or unusual vaginal bleeding, diabetes, multiple sclerosis, migraines, gall-bladder disease, benign breast lumps, endometriosis, epilepsy, any type of heart or circulatory problem including strokes or high blood pressure, kidney or liver disease. (For an alternative approach to the menopause see chapter 9.)

• HOW SAFE ARE TRAVEL VACCINES? •

Let me begin by expressing my profound conviction that not only do vaccinations of any sort not work but they are actively detrimental. Firstly, I have never subscribed to the germ theory. While it makes the drug industry a tremendous amount of money it is totally fallacious and assumes that micro organisms are themselves the main avenue for disease rather than the general health of the host. Secondly, the basic material that goes to make live vaccines is truly disgusting and there are numerous published studies that show that these viruses gobble up large sections of the immune system and can lead to auto-immune diseases such as multiple sclerosis. Thirdly, there are hundreds of thousands of instances where people who have been fully vaccinated have still succumbed to the disease they were supposed to have been protected against. Fourthly, in some unfortunate individuals, vaccines can actually evolve into more serious mutations of the disease in question.

All of this applies just as much to travel vaccines as it does to those given during childhood. My research, for many years now, has taken me all over the world and it is not uncommon for me to visit six or seven countries in a year. Apart from childhood vaccines, which were my mother's decision not mine and over which I had no control, I have never been vaccinated and I have never been ill while travelling. Yet a good read through MIMS, the British doctor's pharmaceutical guide, is enough to make the potential traveller's hair stand on end.

CHOLERA

This is made from the dead form of the organism and where do you think it comes from? Faecal matter! It claims to be effective for six months only. Side-effects, besides serious allergic reactions, can include nerve damage and even mental problems. Besides which the World Health Organisation have now declared the vaccine to be useless. Even MIMS has declared this vaccine 'a public relations gambit'. So why bother?

TYPHOID

Current medical literature acknowledges that there is no satisfactory typhoid vaccine and that protection afforded by the current vaccine is negligible. Give it a miss.

YELLOW FEVER

This is a live vaccine which can cause inflammation of the brain. There are very few places in the word where it is mandatory. When my husband climbed Mount Kilamenjaro in Tanzania, it was suggested but not compulsory, and he came home in thrillingly good health.

POLIO

Polio is now a thing of the past, at least in the Western world, so you may not have any natural antibodies to it. In fact the only new cases of polio in the West are caused by the current polio vaccine. The live vaccine virus is excreted from the mouth and in bowel movements for some weeks after it has been administered. It is therefore very easy to contract the virus when changing the diapers of a baby who has had the vaccine.

TETANUS

The problem with this is that it no longer works well. The vaccine is preserved with a derivative from mercury and, unsurprisingly, some people react very badly to this as mercury in itself is extremely poisonous (see p. 176). It is also known to cause high fever, pain, nerve damage to the inner ear, and anaphylactic shock as well as general deterioration of the nervous system.

MALARIA

I had malaria so many times when I was a little girl in Tanzania that eventually my mother sent me up country to Mbeya to protect me from further attacks. As an adult I have been entirely free of malarial bouts, but as a child I remember being injected with some very powerful anti-malarial drugs. The problem is that most malarial strains are now resistant to chloroquine, the initial anti-malarial pill, and resistance to quinine is on the increase.

All the drugs currently used as a so-called preventive against malaria have toxic side-effects including nausea, severe gastro-intestinal disturbances, vomiting and even psychotic reactions. Extensive high doses of chloroquine can result in damage to the cornea of the eyes or cause tinnitus.

Since the 1970s the Chinese have used Artemisia Annua (Qinghoa) as a very effective anti-malarial treatment with no apparent side-effects. You might like to discuss this with a practitioner qualified in Chinese herbal medicine. As well as this I use a one hundred per cent natural insect repellent which has been successfully tested on Australian soldiers in jungle conditions. Malarial mosquitoes only bite after sun-down so when travelling in malarial zones I cover as much of my body as I can, including my head, and put this lotion on any exposed areas (see Resources Directory). If I can I try to sleep under a mosquito net. With all these precautions I have avoided further bouts of malaria in my adult life, in spite of the fact that insects usually love biting me!

GENERAL ADVICE

So my general advice when travelling abroad is do not have these vaccines and if any one of them is mandatory, don't travel to that country. Harsh, I know, but in the long run very much better for your health. Be sensible about food and water when travelling. Drink water that has been boiled or purified (that includes the water you use to rinse your mouth out after cleaning your teeth). Better to use mineral water which is carbonated in bottles than still water which is more likely to have been filled from a stream in unscrupulous restaurants. Avoid salads, ice-cream, ice-cubes, sorbets and shell-fish, all of which may have come into contact or consist of suspect water. Do not take dairy products which are generally unpasteurised abroad and contain even worse things than they do in the West. Peel all your fruit. Cook all food thoroughly. Wear sandals on the beach, don't walk around bare foot. Swim with your mouth closed. Remember what I said about sewage and sanitary towels and tampons! (see p. 80–82).

The heartening news is ninety-five per cent of all the diseases you can catch abroad are **not** preventable by vaccination and if you're going to a civilised corner of the world (Singapore/Hong Kong/Bali) you're not just endangering your health, you're wasting your money. The one complaint that dominates all travel statistics is diarrhoea. Thirty per cent of those travelling outside Europe or the USA will get it, and of these ninety per cent will sail through it in two days with bed rest and clean water.

APPENDIX 2

• FOOD •

TEMPEH

Tempeh is made of fermented whole soya beans, and like tofu it is low in fat and calories but much more full of flavour. Sold in the refrigerator section of health food stores it looks like a solid creamy white cake and once bought needs to be stored in the refrigerator and eaten within a week. It freezes quite well and can be stored for two to three months.

TOFU

Tofu is also readily available in health food stores and because it tastes so neutral it will absorb a wide variety of flavours. It can be baked, dried, grilled, marinated, scrambled, liquidised and turned in cream, steamed or crumbled. It comes in two forms: as a solid white block which can be stored in the refrigerator at home for up to a week provided the water is changed daily to help keep it fresh, or as soft tofu in a packet from which it needs to be squeezed out. Firm tofu is best for cooking, stir frying and crumbling whilst soft tofu makes excellent sauces, dips and dressings. Tofu is very rich in calcium and weight for weight contains more calcium than dairy milk. It is also high in iron, magnesium, phosphorus, sodium and potassium and essential B vitamins as well as vitamin E. As a protein it is alkaline rather than acid so combines well with starches.

QUINOA

Quinoa is an interesting grain which is increasingly appearing in natural health food stores. It looks rather like large yellow mustard seeds and if toasted tastes nutty. It needs to be rinsed well in hot water before using because of the saponin that covers it and protects it from insects and birds.

TVP

TVP stands for texturised vegetable protein and is manufactured from soya beans in granule form. Once soaked in hot water it looks remarkably like mincemeat. It is often fortified with vitamin B12 and as I suspect this vitamin is synthetically made I tend to avoid it (see p. 23). The mince or chunks taste better if you sauté them in a little water and olive oil before re-hydrating them further. TVP is also found in manufactured vegetarian burgers and sausages which can be purchased from the freeze cabinet of supermarkets and in health food stores.

QUORN

Quorn is a distant relative of the mushroom and is grown in a fermenter. It is a good halfway step to moving through vegetarianism on to veganism. (It contains egg white as well as vegetable flavouring.) It absorbs flavours well so is ideal for marinading and is widely available in ready-made chill-cook meals like pies, curries and stir frys.

LINSEED

Organic linseed is available from health food shops.

APPENDIX 3

———

• SLANT BOARD EXERCISES •

To perform these exercises, one end of the slant board should be elevated to a height of about 12″ while the other should remain firmly on the ground. You should lie on the slant board so that your feet are at the elevated end.

1. Lie on your back on the board with your arms by your sides for at least 10 minutes. This will allow gravity to help your abdominal organs to get into their positions.
2. Raise your arms directly above your head, making your body into a straight line. This exercise stretches your abdomen. Repeat this exercise 10 to 15 times; this will stretch the abdominal muscles and pull the abdomen towards the shoulders.
3. While holding your breath, move your abdominal organs towards your shoulders, by contracting the abdominal muscles, then allowing them to relax. Repeat this exercise 10 to 15 times.
4. Pat your abdomen vigorously with both hands. then lean first to the left side and then the right side, each time patting the stretched side 10 to 15 times each. Using your abdominal muscles, bring your body to the sitting position, then return to the lying position. If possible, do this 3 times. Then lie down flat and roll a ball around the abdomen, pressing deeply and following the shape of the colon from left to right.
5. Bend your knees, and raise your legs at the hips, drawing them towards your chest. While in this position turn your head from side to side 5 or 6 times, then lift your head slightly and rotate 3 or 4 times.
6. Lift your legs so they are almost at right angles to your body. Make outward circular movements 8 or 10 times. Increase to 25 movements after a week or two of exercising.
7. Bend your knees. Straighten one leg and raise it slowly about 10″ from the slant board, keeping your back firmly on the board. Repeat 10 times, then change legs.
8. Raise your legs in the air and make circular movements as if you were riding a bicycle. Do this 14 to 25 times.

When you have finished you slant board exercises, relax and rest, letting the blood circulate in your head for 10 minutes.

RESOURCE DIRECTORY

• ASSOCIATIONS AND SCHOOLS •

The British Institute of Homeopathy
520 Washington Blvd., Suite 423
Marina Del Ray, CA 90292
Phone (310) 335-1205
Fax (310) 827-5766

The Council of Colleges of Acupuncture and Oriental Medicine
1424 16th St. NW
Suite 501
Washington, D.C. 20036

European Herbal Alliance of which Kitty Campion is the treasurer will supply a list of fully qualified herbal practitioners trained by Kitty Campion of the College of Herbs and Natural Healing, or with the National Institute of Herbal Medicine, or the General Council and Register of Consultant Medical Herbalists. Write to Kevin Embling-Evans:
18 Sussex Square
Brighton
BN2 5AA
England

Manual Lymphatic Drainage Association
8 Wittenham Lane
Dorchester on Thames
Oxon
OX10 7JW England
Phone 01865 340385

National Center for Homeopathy
801 N. Fairfax Street
Suite 306
Alexandria, VA 22314
Phone (703) 548-7790

The New England School of Acupuncture
30 Common Street
Watertown, MA 02172
Phone (617) 926-4271

Pacific Institute of Oriental Medicine
12 West 27th Street, 9th Floor
New York, NY 10001
Phone (212) 685-3456

The School of Natural Healing (Founded by Dr Christopher)
P.O. Box 412
Springville, UT 84663
Phone (800) 372-8255

• COLONIC TREATMENT •

Ultimate Trends
P.O. Box 1427
Sandy, UT 84091
Phone (800) 468-3416

• DETOXIFIERS •

Flora Inc.
Phone (800) 446-2110

Pronatura, Inc.
6211-A West Howard Street
Niles, IL 60714
Phone (800) 555-7580

Zand Herbal
P.O. Box 2039
Boulder, CO 80306
Phone (303) 786-8558

• ENVIRONMENTAL PRODUCTS •

Pesticide Remover
Allens Naturally
P.O. Box 514
Farmington, MI 48332-0514

Allens has a Fruit and Veggie Wash for removing chemicals from produce.

Propolis
Montana Naturals International, Inc.
19994 Highway 93
Arlee, MT 59821
Phone (800) 872-7218

Montana Naturals carries bee pollen, royal jelly, propolis and energy formulas containing ginkgo and ginseng.

Wholistic Research Company
Brighthaven
Robin's Lane
Lolworth
Cambridge CB3 8HH
Phone 01954 781074

Particularly knowledgeable about ELF reduction and VDUs. Supplier of day-light simulation light bulbs and other useful information about SAD syndrome, including contacts for equipment. Supplier of douche and enema kits. The company also supplies Philips Daylight Blue and Sungrolite lightbulbs, both of which provide light which more closely approaches that of daylight, enhancing visual accuracy and making reading easier. Supplier of wheatgrass juice press and reverse osmosis water filters.

• FEMININE PRODUCTS •

Alvin Last, Inc.
19 Babcock Place
Yonkers, NY 10701
Phone (800) 527-8422

Alvin Last has a vaginal moisturizing gel made with wild yam extract and vitamin E.

Glad Rags
P.O. Box 1275
Portland, OR 97212
Phone (800) 799-4523

Glad Rags has soft cotton chamois pads which snap around your underwear and stay in place. They are in the process (at the time of publication) of developing organic diapers.

Mountain Rose Herbs
P.O. Box 2000H
Redway, CA 95560
Phone (800) 879-3337
Mountain Rose Herb has teas, herbs, oils, lotions, soaps and feminine pads.

Natracare
191 University Blvd., Suite 294
Denver, CO 80206
web site http://www.indra.com/natracare

Natracare has all-cotton tampons, panty shields and pads.

Skin Brushes
Loofa Brite
P.O. Box 246
New Paltz, NY 12561

• HERBS, ESSENTIAL OILS AND FLOWER ESSENCES •

Bioforce of America LTD.
Kinderhook, NY 12106
Phone (800) 445-8802

Bioforce UK Limited
Olympic Business Park
Dundonald
Ayrshire
KA2 9BE England
Phone 01563 851177

I have dealt with this company now for many years and greatly admire the fact that by and large they are unique among herbal manufacturers for using only freshly harvested herbs in their tinctures. The herbs are cultivated in a remote north-eastern corner of Switzerland between 800 to 1500 feet above sea level which encourages the condensation of the healing properties in them. In other words they have to be hardy and powerful to survive at this height. This company is also particularly strict about harvesting according to strict protocols. For example, echinacea purpurea is harvested when it reaches three to four feet in height when fifty per cent of the flowers are in bloom and fifty per cent in bud. Harvesting takes place after midday.

While many professional herbalists in practice, including myself, are particularly keen to harvest their own herbs freshly whenever possible, most commercially available herbal tinctures are not manufactured to Bioforce's particularly high standards. All Bioforce's products are readily available in health food shops.

Daniele Ryman's Essential Oils can be purchased by mail order by writing to her at the
Daniele Ryman Clinic
Park Lane Hotel
Piccadilly
London W1Y 8BX
England
Phone 171 7536708

Flower Essence Society
P.O. Box 459
Nevada City, CA 95959
Phone (800) 548-0075
Fax (916) 265-6467
E-mail fes@nccn.net

Hard-to-Find Herbalware
6715 Donerail Drive
Sacramento, CA 95842

Herb Research Foundation
1007 Peral St., Suite 200
Boulder, CO 80302
Phone (800) 748-2617

Nature's Plus
548 Broadhollow Road
Melville, NY 11747

Nature's Plus has herbs, digestive enzymes and spirulina. All their products are tested by third parties.

Nature's Way Products, Inc.
10 Mountain Springs Parkway
Springville, UT 84663

Nature's Way has a wide selection of products ranging from capsules, Femaprin to cayenne supplements, ginkgo biloba and more.

A Nelson & Company Limited
5 Endeavour Way
Wimbledon
London
SW19 9UE
England
Phone 0181 946 8527

Makes a superb range of herbal ointments and creams. I particularly like this company because they use, as Bioforce does, as much fresh base herbs as they can. Scientific testing using chromatography proves that fresh herb preparations contain more of the active constituents and are more stable compared to their counterparts manufactured from dried herbs.

Oshahadi
P.O. Box 824
Rogers, AR 72757
Phone (501) 636-0579
Fax (501) 636-3785

Solgar Vitamin and Herb Company, Inc.
500 Willow Tree Road
Leonia, NJ 07605
web site http://www.solgar. com

Solgar has over 400 products including digestive enzymes, vitamins, minerals and herbs. This company supplies Earth Source, a good combination of many of the superfoods, together with single herbs and combination formulas which are grown and processed to an extremely high standard and mainly packed in vegetarian capsules.

• HOME KITS •

Kitty Campion
25 Curzon street
Basford
Newcastle-under-Lyme
Staffordshire
ST5 9PD
Phone 01782 711592

Supplier of T-tree pessaries, skin brushes, douche and enema kits and most of the composite herbal formulas mentioned in this book. Also supplier of Nature's Superfoods which contains most of the ingredients mentioned on pages 25-32.

Femina Cones (for testing and strengthening of pelvic floor muscles) are available from:
Colgate Medical Limited
1 Fairacres Estate
Dedworth Road
Windsor
Berkshire
SL4 4LE
England
Phone 01753 860378

• HOW TO FIND A PRACTITIONER •

New Age Journal Online
http://www.newage.com/home/newage/

Natural Medicine, Complementary Health Care and Alternative Therapies
http://www.amrta.org/~amrta

National Commission for the Certification of Acupuncturists (NCCA)
1424 16th St. NW
Suite 501
Washington, D.C. 20036

• MERCURY-FREE DENTISTRY •

Jack Levenson
1 Welbeck House
62 Welbeck Street
London
W1N 7SB
England
Phone 0171 486 3127

• NUTRITION AND NUTRITIONAL RESEARCH •

The British Society for Nutritional Medicine
5 Somerhill Road
Hove
East Sussex
BN3 1RP
England
This society is interested in the effects of food on health.

Herbal Teas
Celestial Seasonings
4600 Sleepytime Drive
Boulder, CO 80301-3292
Phone (303) 530-5300

Traditional Medicinals
4515 Ross Road
Sebastopol, CA 95472
Phone (707) 823-8911

Natural Food Store
Sweet Pea Natural Foods
Rt. 100
Waitsfield, VT 05673
Phone (802) 496-7763

Sweet Pea has a wide selection of natural and organic products and a very knowledgeable staff. They will ship anywhere in the US. Call for more information.

Organic Wines
Chartrand Imports
P.O. Box 1319
Rockland, ME 04841
Phone (207) 594-7300

Fitzpatrick Winery
BW 4978
Somerset, CA 95684
(916) 620-3248

• SUPERFOODS •

Bioflavonoids
Nature's Answer, Inc.
Dept. D8 75 Commerce Drive
Hauppauge, NY 11788
Phone (800) 645-5720

Juicer for Wheat Grass
Perfect Health
Dept. BN
5423 Driftwood Street
Oxnard, CA 93035
Phone (805) 382-2021

Spirulina, Wheatgerm and Flaxseed Oils
Nature's Plus
548 Broadhollow Road
Melville, NY 11747

Spectrum Naturals
133 Copeland Street
Petaluma, CA 94952

Earthrise Company
P.O. Box 60-CA5
Petaluma, CA 94953
web site http://www.earthrise.com

ADDITIONAL RESOURCES

BIBLIOGRAPHY

Airola, P., *Everywoman's Book,* Contemporary Books, Chicago, IL, 1984.

Christopher, J., *Every Woman's Herbal,* Dr. Chris Publications, Springville, Utah, 1994.

Diamond H. and M., *Fit for Life II,* Bantam Books, New York, NY, 1993.

Griggs, B., *Green Pharmacy, Inner Traditions, Rochester, VT, 1991.*

Harrison, J., *Love Your Disease,* Hay House, Inc., Carson City, CA, 1988.

Jacobson, M. et al., *Safe Food,* Living Planet Press, Washington, D.C., 1991.

Jensen, B. and Anderson, M., *Empty Harvest,* Avery Publishing Group Inc., New York, NY, 1993.

Klaper, M., *Vegan Nutrition: Pure and Simple,* Gentle World, Inc., Alachua, FL, 1987.

McIntyre, A., *The Complete Woman's Herbal,* Henry Holt & Co., Inc., New York, NY, 1995.

McIntyre, A., *Herbal Medicine,* Charles E. Tuttle Co., Inc., Boston, MA, 1993.

Robbins, J., *Diet for a New America,* Stillpoint Publishing, Walpole, NH, 1987.

Medical Glossary

---

agoraphobia	fear of open spaces
allergen	a substance which provokes an allergic response
amenorrhea	lack of menstruation
anaemia	lack of haemgloblin in the blood
angina pectoris	heart disease manifested by chest pain or exertion
anorexia	self-starvation
anxiety	nervous disorder characterised by a state of excessive uneasiness
bartholin cysts	cysts which form as a result of the infection of the Bartholin glands (situated just outside the vaginal opening)
bulimia	eating and vomiting cycles
cancer	malignant growths which invade healthy tissue and destroy it, often spreading to other parts of the body unchecked by the immune system
candida albicans	a fungal infection which commonly affect the vagina but may also affect other areas (such as the inside of the mouth or intestine)
cervical erosion	where the cells which normally occur in the inner lining cervix appear on the outside causing redness, excessive production of mucus and sometimes bleeding
chilblains	itchy, red swelling caused by impaired blood supply and poor circulation
chlamydia	trachomatic micro-organisms which can affect cells in the cervix, bladder of fallopian tubes
claustrophobia	dread of confined spaces
colitis	inflammation of the colon
constipation	infrequent bowel movements
cystitis	bacterial infection of the bladder
delirium tremens (DTs)	result of coming off high alcohol intake abruptly
depression	mental illness
diarrhoea	where the colon becomes irritated and goes into overdrive
diverticulitis	where a weakness in the colon wall caused the development of infected pouches (diverticula)
dysmenorrhoea	difficult and painful menstruation

dyspepsia	indigestion
endometriosis	tissue which normally lines the uterus found in other parts of the body
fibroids	hard, lumpy, non-malignant growths of smooth muscle and fibrous connective tissue
haemorrhoids	engorged veins inside or outside the anus
hiccups	an involuntary spasms of the diaphragm and vocal cords
hyperactivity	an abnormally active person (usually child)
hypertension	high blood pressure
hyperventilation	overbreathing
hypoglycaemia	low blood sugar
incontinence	inability to retain urine
indigestion	burning pain or discomfort on eating
insomnia	inability to sleep
irritable bowel syndrome	nervous spasmodic colon
kidney stones	calcareous growths in the kidneys
leaky gut syndrome	increased gut permeability
leucorrhoea	excessive white vaginal discharge
metrorrhagia	uterine haemorrhage outside of normal menstruation
migraine	recurrent headaches with visual and/or gastrointestinal disturbance
miscarriage	loss of a foetus usually between the 12th and 28th week of pregnancy
nightmares	bad dreams
oedema	water retention and consequent swelling just before menstruation
osteoporosis	thinning of the bones
pelvic inflammatory disease	inflammation of the womb, fallopian tubes and ovaries
phlebitis	inflammation of a vein, often accompanied by blood clots
polyps	growths from the endometrium lining of cervical canal
post viral fatigue syndrome	a malfunctioning immune system with one or several consecutive viruses
premenstrual syndrome	symptoms experienced before menstruation
pubic lice	small blood-sucking insects which burrow into the skin
salpingitis	acute of chronic inflammation of the fallopian tubes
thrombosis	clots in the blood stream which block a vessel or travel as emboli around the circulation system and lodge elsewhere
toothache	aching in the tooth or gums due to localised infection
travel sickness	nausea while travelling
trichomoniasis	parastic infection around the anus or vagina
ulcers	inflammation of stomach or duodenal lining
varicose veins	engorged veins
warts, genital	viral infection of genital area

Glossary of Herbs

Aconite, *Aconitum napellus*
Agrimony, *Agrimonia enpatoria*
Alfalfa, *Medicago sativa*
Allspice, *Pimento officinalis*
Almond, *Amygdalus communis*
Aloe, *Aloe vera*
Angelica, *Angelica archangelica*
Anise, *Pimpinella anisum*
Aniseed, *Pimpinella anisum*
Arnica, *Arnice montana*
Arrowroot, *Maranta arundinaceae*
Artichoke, *Cynara scolymus*
Ash, *Fraxinus excelsior*
Autumn crocus, *Colchicum autumnale*

Balm, Lemon, *Melissa officinalis*
Balm of Gilead, *Populus gileadensis*
Barley, *Hordeum distichon*
Basil, *Ocimum basilicum*
Bay Laurel, *Laurel nobilis*
Bayberry, *Myrica cerifera*
Bearberry, *Arctostaphylos ulva-ursi*
Belladonna, *Atrope belladonna*
Benzoin, *Styrax benzion*
Bergamot, *Monarda didyma*
Beth Root, *Trillium pendulum*
Betony (Wood), *Stachys betonica*
Bilberry, *Vaccinium myrtillus*
Birch, *Betula alba*
Black cohosh, *Cimicifuga racemose*
Black horehound, *Ballota nigra*
Black walnut, *Juglans nigra*
Blessed thistle, *Cnicus benedictus*
Blue cohosh, *Caulophyllum thalictroides*

Blue flag, *Iris versicolor*
Blue rue, *Ruta graveolens*
Boneset, *Eupatroium perfoliatum*
Brooklime, *Veronica beccabunga*
Borage, *Borago officinalis*
Bramble, *Rubus fructicosus*
Broom, *Cytisus scoparius*
Buchu, *Barosma betulina*
Buckwheat, *Fagopyrum esculentum*
Buckthorn, *Rhamnus cathartica*
Burdock, *Arctium lappe*
Butterbur, *Petasites vulgaris*
Buttercup, *Ranunculus bulbosus*
Bryony (white), *Byronia dioica*

Calamus, *Acorus calumus*
Camphor, *Cinnamonum camphora*
Cape Aloes, *Aloe ferox*
Caster oil plant, *Ricinus communis*
Caraway, *Carum carvl cardamon*
Carrot (Wild), *Daucus corote*
Cascara sagrada, *Rhamnus purshianus*
Castor oil plant, *Ricinus communis*
Catnip, *Nepeta cataria*
Cayenne, *Capsicum minimum*
Celandine (greater), *Chelidonium majus*
Celery, *Apium graveolens*
Chamomile (common), *Matricaria chamomilla*
Chamomile (German), *Anthemis nobills*
Chaparrel, *Larrea divaricate cav*
Chasterberries, *Angus castus*
Chestnut (horse), *Aesculus hippocastanum*
Chevril, *Anthriscus cerefolium*
Chickweed, *Stellaria media*
Chicory, *Cichorium intybus*
Chive, *Allum scloanoprasum*
Cicely (Sweet), *Myrrhis odorate*
Cinnamon, *Cinnamonum zeylanicum*
Clary sage, *Salvia horminoides*
Cleavers, *Gallum aparine*
Clove, *Eugenia caryophyllata*
Clover (red), *Trifolium pratense*
Coltsfoot, *Tussilaga farfare*
Comfrey, *Symphytum officinale*
Cornflower, *Centaurea cyanus*

Cornsilk, *Zea mays*
Couch grass, *Agropyrum repens*
Cowslip, *Primula veris*
Cramp bark, *Viburnum opulus*
Cranberry, *Vaccinum macrocarpon*
Cucumber, *Cucumis sativa*
Cudweed marsh, *Ghaphalium uliginosum*
Currant (red), *Ribes rubrum*

Daisy, *Bellis perennis*
Damiana, *Damiana aphrodisiaca*
Dandelion, *Taraxacum officinale*
Dill, *Anethum graveolens*
Dock (yellow), *Rumex, crispus*
Dulse, *Fucus vesiculosis*
Echinacea, *Echinacea angustifolia*
Elderberry, *Sambucus nigra*
Elecampagne, *Inula relenlum*
Elm (Slippery), *Ulmus fulva*
Eucalyptus, *Eucalyptus globulus*
Primrose (Evening), *Oenothera biennis*
Eyebright, *Euphrasia officinalis*

Fennel, *Foeniculum vulgare*
Fenugreek, *Trigonella foenum-graecum*
Feverfew, *Chrysanthemum parthenium*
Figwort (Knotted), *Scrophularia nodosa*
Flax, *Linum usitatissimum*
Foxglove, *Digitalis purpurea*
Fumitory, *Fumaria officinalis*

Garlic, *Allium sativum*
Gentlan, *Gentiana*
Gentian (yellow), *Gentiana lutca*
Geranium, *Geranium maculatum*
Ginger (Root), *Zingiber officinale*
Ginseng:
    Asiatic, *Panax ginseng*
    Siberian, *Eleutherococcus senticosus*
Goat's rue, *Galega officinalis*
Goldenseal, *Hydrastis canadensis*
Gotu Kola, *Hydrocotyle asiatica*
Grape root (Oregon), *Berberis aquifolium*
Gravel root, *Eupatorium purpureum*
Grindella, *Grindelia camporium, Grindelia cuneifolla, Grindelia squarrose*

Groundsel, *Senicio viscosus*
Gypsy weed (Bugie Weed, *Lycopus europaeus*

Hawthorn, *Crataegus monogyna*
Heartsease, *Viola tricolor*
Heather, *Calluna vulgaris*
Hibiscus (red), *Rosa-Sinensis*
Hellebore (faise), *Adonis autumnalis*
Hemlock, *Conium maculatum*
Henna, *Lawsonia alba*
Holly, *illex aquifolium*
Honeysuckle, *Lonicera caprifolium*
Hops, *Humulus lupulus*
Horehound, Marrubium vulgare
Horse Radish, *Cochlearia armoracle*
Horsetail, *Equisetum*
Houseleek, *Sempervivum tectorum*
Hydrangea (root), *Hydrangea arborescens*
Hyssop, *Hyssopus officinalis*

Ipecac, *Cephaelis ipecacuanha*
Iris, *Iris versicolor*
Ivy (ground), *Glechoma hederacea*

Jasmine (general), *Jasminum*
Juniper, *Juniperus communis*

Kava Kava, *Piper methysticum*
Kelp, *Fucus vesiculosus*

Lady's Mantle, *Alchamilla vulgaris*
Lady's Slipper, *Cypripedium pubescens*
Lavender, *Santolina*
Cotton Lavender, *Chamaecy parissum*
English Lavender, *Lavandula vera*
Lemon, *Citrus limonum*
Lemon balm, *Melissa officinalis*
Lettuce, *Lactuce virosa*
Lilly (White Water), *Nymphaea odorata*
Lime, *Citrus acida*
Linseed (flax), *Linum usitatissimum*
Liquorice, *Glycyrrhiza glabra*
Lobelia, *Lobelia inflata*
Loosestrife (purple), *Lythrum salicaria*
Lovage, *Levisticum officinale*

Lungwort, *Sticta pulmonaria*
Lupin, *Leguminosae*

Malefern, *Dryopteris feliz-mas*
Mandrake, *Atropa mandragora*
Marigold, *Calendula officinalis*
Marjoram:
    (sweet), *Origanum marjorana*
    (wild), *Origanum vulgare*
Meadowsweet, *Fllipendula ulmarie*
Mimosa, *Mimosa fragigolia*
Mint (Spear), *Mentha viridis*
Mistletoe, *Viscum album*
Moss (Icelandic), *Cetraria islandica*
Moss (Irish), *Chondrus crispus*
Moss (Sphagnum), *Sphagnum cymbifolium*
Motherwort, *Leonurus cardiaca*
Mugworth, *Artemisia vulgaris*
Mullein, *Verbascum thapsus*
Mustard:
    (black), *Brassica nigra*
    (white), *Brassica alba*
Myrrh, *Commiphora myrrha*

Nasturtium, *Tropaeolum majus*
Neroli (Orange), *Citrus aurantium*
Nettles, *Urticaceae*
Nutmeg, *Myristica fragrans*

Oak, *Lavercus robur*
Oats, *Avena sativa*
Olive, *Olea europaea*
Onion, *Allium cepe*
Orange:
    (bitter), *Citrus vulgaris*
    (sweet), *Citrus aurantium*
Orchard (Wild), *Orchid masculata*
Oregon Grape Root, *Berberis aqulfolium*
Origanum, *Ulgare aureum*
Orris Root, *Iris florentia*
Pansy, *Viola tricolor*
Parsley, *Petroselinum sativum*
Passion flower, *Anemone pusatilla*
Pan d'arco (Taheebo), *Tabenia impetiginosa*
Peach, *Prunus persica*

Pellitory of the Wall, *Parletaria officinalis*
Penny Royal, *Mentha pulegium*
Peppermint, *Mentha piperita*
Periwinkle (Greater), *Vinca major*
Pilewort, *Ranunculus ficaria*
Pine, *Pinacaes*
Plaintain, *Plantago major*
Pleurisy root, *Asclepias tuberose*
Poke root, *Phytolacca decandra*
Pomegranate, *Punica granatum*
Poppys:
   (Red), *Papaver rhoeas*
   (White), *Papaver somniferum*
Prickly ash, *Xanthoxylum americanum*
Primrose, *Primula vulgaris*
Privet, *Liqustrum vulgare*
Psyltium, *Plantago psyllium*
Pulsatilla, *Anemone pulsatilla*
Purslane:
   (green), *Portulaca oleracea*
   (golden), *Portulaca sative*

Quassia (bark), *Picraena exceisa*
Quince, *Pyrus cydonia*

Raspberry, *Rubus idaaus*
Rest-harrow, *Ononis arvensis*
Rhubarb (Turkey), *Rheum palmatum*
Rose, *Rosecaes*
Rosehip, *Rosa canina*
Rosemary, *Rosemarinus officinalis*
Rue, *Ruta graveolens*

Sage, *Salvia officinalis*
Sandalwood (Yellow), *Santalum album*
Sassafras, *Sassafras officinale*
Savory:
   (summer), *Saturela hortensis*
   (winter), *Saturela montano*
Saw Palmetto, *Sarenoa serrulata*
Scabious, (Field) *Scabiosa arvensis*
Scullcap (Virquinian), *Scutellaria lateriflora*
Seaweed (general), *Fucus vesiculosis*
Self-heal, *Prunella vulgaris*
Senna, *Cassia acutifolia*

Shepherd's Purse, *Capsella burse-pastoris*
Skunk cabbage, *Symplocar pus foctidus*
Soap wort, *Saponaria officinalis*
Solomon's Seal, *Polygonatium multiflorum*
Sorrel:
    (French), *Rumex scatatus*
    (garden), *Rumex acetosa*
Southernwood, *Field artemisla campestria*
Speedwell, *Common veronica officinalis*
Squaw Vine, *Mitchella repens*
Squill, *Urginea scilla*
St John's Wort, *Hypericum perforatum*
Stillingia, *Stillingia sylvatica*
Stone root, *Collinsonia canadensis*
Strawberry, *Frangaria vesca*
Sumac mooth, *Rhus glabie*
Sunflower, *Helianthus annvus*

Tansy, *Tanacetum vulgare*
Tea tree, *Melalenca alternifolia*
Thuja, *Thuja occidentalis*
Thyme:
    (garden), *Thymus vulgaris*
    (wild), *Thymus serpyllum*
Toad flax, *Linaria vulgaris*
Tobacco, *Nicotlana tabacum*
Tormentil, *Potentilla tormentilla*
Tumeric, *Curcuma longa*

Unicorn (False), *Chamaelirlum luteum*
Unicorn (True), *Aletris farinosa*
Uva-Ursi, *Arctostaphylos ulva-ursi*

Valerian, *Valeriana officinalis*
Vervain (blue), *Verbena officinalis*
Vine (general), *Vitis vinifera*
Violet (sweet), *Viola odorata*

Watercress, *Nasturtium officinale*
Willow (white), *Salix alba*
Wild indigo, *Baptisia tunctoria*
Willow-herb (Rosebay), *Epilobium angustifolium*
Winter green, *Gaultheria procumbens*
Witch hazel, *Hamamelis virginiana*
Woodruff, *Asperula odorate*

Wormwood (Common), Artemisia absinthium

Yam (Wild), *Dioscorea villosa*
Yarrow, *Archillea millefolium*

Index